Kunio Shirato (Ed.)
Venous Thromboembolism
Prevention and Treatment

K. Shirato (Ed.)

Venous Thromboembolism

Prevention and Treatment

With 44 Figures, Including 9 in Color

Springer

Kunio Shirato, M.D., Ph.D.
Professor
Department of Cardiovascular Medicine
Tohoku University Graduate School of Medicine
1-1 Seiryo-machi, Aoba-ku, Sendai 980-8574, Japan

Library of Congress Control Number: 2004113935

ISBN 4-431-22080-1 Springer-Verlag Tokyo Berlin Heidelberg New York

Springer is a part of Springer Science+Business Media
springeronline.com

Printed in Japan

Typesetting: SNP Best-set Typesetter Ltd., Hong Kong
Printing and binding: Shinano, Inc., Japan

Printed on acid-free paper

Preface

The fact that pulmonary thromboembolism is still associated with a high rate of mortality in Japan has led to the International Symposium for Pulmonary Thromboembolism being held regularly in the country. The first was convened in 1998 in Yokkaichi, Mie, as the International Symposium on Pulmonary Embolism. This was organized by Professor T. Nakano and Professor S.Z. Goldhaber and the proceedings were published by Springer-Verlag, Tokyo, under the title *Pulmonary Embolism*. The second was held in 2000 in Chiba as the Millennium Symposium on Pulmonary Thromboembolism. This event was under the auspices of Professor N. Nakajima and Professor T. Kuriyama. Most recently, this commemorative book has been compiled, based on the International Symposium on Pulmonary Thromboembolism, held in Sendai on November 2, 2003.

This collection of work from specialists in the field addresses certain features specific to Japan in terms of epidemiological analysis, the treatment of pulmonary thromboembolism, traveler's thrombosis, and the prevention of deep vein thromboembolism, the latter being a possible direct cause of pulmonary thromboembolism.

As you may notice after reading this book, there are some differences between conditions in Japan and in Western countries, particularly in treatment selection and prevention of the disease. For example, in Japan, inferior vena cava filters tend to be used frequently, and percutaneous cardiopulmonary support, or PCPS, is applied without hesitation to treat patients in a serious condition.

We realize that the clinical skill level in Japan for treating pulmonary thromboembolism must catch up with that in the West, and we believe that a different approach to treatment selection could result in new evidence and, ultimately, in progress in the medical treatment of this disease.

My deepest thanks go to the contributors, the senior members of Tohoku University's First Department of Internal Medicine, and the fellows of the

Department of Cardiovascular Medicine, who have all helped make this book the valuable resource that it is.

Kunio Shirato
Department of Cardiovascular Medicine
Tohoku University Graduate School of Medicine
Sendai, Japan

Contributors to the International Symposium on Pulmonary Thromboembolism 2003, and to this book:

Jun Demachi, M.D.
Noriko Kakudo, M.D.
Jun Nawata, M.D.
Hiroki Ohtani, M.D.
Minako Oikawa, M.D.
Boon-Hooi Ong, M.D.
Kenya Saji, M.D.
Masahito Sakuma, M.D.
Koichiro Sugimura, M.D.
Jun Suzuki, M.D.
Tohru Takahashi, M.D.
Huan Wang, M.D.
Rika Kobayashi (secretary)
Mayumi Sugimura (secretary)

Contents

Authors

Adnet, F.
SAMU 93, UPRES 34-09, Hôpital Avicenne
125, Rue de Stalingrad, 93009, Bobigny, France

Aklog, Lishan
Department of Cardiothoracic Surgery, Mount Sinai Medical Center
1190 Fifth Avenue, 1028, New York, NY, USA

Ando, Motomi
Department of Cardiovascular Surgery, Fujita Health University School of Medicine
1-98 Dengakugakubo, Kutsukake-cho, Toyoake, Aichi 470-1192, Japan

Belcaro, Gianni
Department of Biomedical Sciences, IRVINE2 Vascular Lab, Chieti University, and San Valentino Vascular Screening Project (Pe)
Via Vespucci 65, 65100 Pescara, Italy

Böttiger, Bernd W.
Department of Anaesthesiology, University of Heidelberg
Im Neuenheimer Field 110, D-69120 Heidelberg, Germany

Catineau, J.
SAMU 93, UPRES 34-09, Hôpital Avicenne
125, Rue de Stalingrad, 93009, Bobigny, France

Cesarone, Maria Rosaria
Department of Biomedical Sciences, IRVINE2 Vascular Lab, Chieti University, and San Valentino Vascular Screening Project (Pe)
Via Vespucci 65, 65100 Pescara, Italy

Demachi, Jun
Department of Cardiovascular Medicine, Tohoku University Graduate School of Medicine
1-1 Seiryo-machi, Aoba-ku, Sendai 980-8574, Japan

Dugall, Mark
Department of Biomedical Sciences, IRVINE2 Vascular Lab, Chieti University, and San Valentino Vascular Screening Project (Pe)
Via Vespucci 65, 65100 Pescara, Italy

Errichi, Bruno M.
Department of Biomedical Sciences, IRVINE2 Vascular Lab, Chieti University, and San Valentino Vascular Screening Project (Pe)
Via Vespucci 65, 65100 Pescara, Italy

Fujita, Satoru
Department of Orthopaedic Surgery, Takarazuka Daiichi Hospital
19-5 Kogetsu-cho, Takarazuka, Hyogo 665-0832, Japan

Hamersley, Sheri Lynn
15005 Shady Grove Road Ste 340, Rockville, MD 20850, USA

Hata, Yasushi
Department of Surgery and Clinical Oncology, Graduate School of Medicine, Osaka University
E2, 2-2 Yamadaoka, Suita, Osaka 565-0871, Japan

Hoshino, Ryo
Department of Cardiovascular Surgery, Fujita Health University School of Medicine
1-98 Dengakugakubo, Kutsukake-cho, Toyoake, Aichi 470-1192, Japan

Hull, Russell D.
University of Calgary, 601 South Tower, Foothills Hospital
1403-29 Street NW, Calgary, Alberta, T2N2T9, Canada

Ikeda, Masataka
Department of Surgery and Clinical Oncology, Graduate School of Medicine, Osaka University
E2, 2-2 Yamadaoka, Suita, Osaka 565-0871, Japan

Kakkar, Ajay K.
Centre for Surgical Sciences, Barts and The London School for Medicine and Dentistry, and Thrombosis Research Institute
Emmanuel Kaye Building, Manresa Road, London SW3 6LR, UK

Kakudo, Noriko
Department of Cardiovascular Medicine, Tohoku University Graduate School of Medicine
1-1 Seiryo-machi, Aoba-ku, Sendai 980-8574, Japan

Kobayashi, Takao
Shinshu University School of Health Sciences
3-1-1 Asahi, Matsumoto, Nagano 390-8621, Japan

Konstantinides, Stavros
Department of Cardiology and Pulmonary Medicine, Georg August University
Robert Koch Strasse 40, D-37075 Goettingen, Germany

Lapostolle, F.
SAMU 93, UPRES 34-09, Hôpital Avicenne
125 Rue de Stalingrad, 93009 Bobigny, France

Ledda, Andrea
Department of Biomedical Sciences, IRVINE2 Vascular Lab, Chieti University, and San Valentino Vascular Screening Project (Pe)
Via Vespucci 65, 65100 Pescara, Italy

Monden, Morito
Department of Surgery and Clinical Oncology, Graduate School of Medicine, Osaka University
E2, 2-2 Yamadaoka, Suita, Osaka 565-0871, Japan

Morio, Hiroshi
Department of Internal Medicine, Narita Red Cross Hospital
90-1 Iida-cho, Narita, Chiba 286-8523, Japan

Nawata, Jun
Department of Cardiovascular Medicine, Tohoku University Graduate School of Medicine
1-1 Seiryo-machi, Aoba-ku, Sendai 980-8574, Japan

Niwa, Akihiro
Department of Cardiology, Musashino Red Cross Hospital
1-26-1 Kyonan-cho, Musashino, Tokyo 180-8610, Japan

Ong, Boon-Hooi
Department of Cardiovascular Medicine, Tohoku University Graduate School of Medicine
1-1 Seiryo-machi, Aoba-ku, Sendai 980-8574, Japan

Pineo, Graham F.
University of Calgary, 601 South Tower, Foothills Hospital
1403-29 Street NW, Calgary, Alberta, T2N2T9, Canada

Saji, Kenya
Department of Cardiovascular Medicine, Tohoku University Graduate School of Medicine
1-1 Seiryo-machi, Aoba-ku, Sendai 980-8574, Japan

Sakon, Masato
Department of Surgery and Clinical Oncology, Graduate School of Medicine, Osaka University
E2, 2-2 Yamadaoka, Suita, Osaka 565-0871, Japan

Sakuma, Masahito
Department of Cardiovascular Medicine, Tohoku University Graduate School of Medicine
1-1 Seiryo-machi, Aoba-ku, Sendai 980-8574, Japan

Sato, Masato
Department of Cardiovascular Surgery, Fujita Health University School of Medicine
1-98 Dengakugakubo, Kutsukake-cho, Toyoake, Aichi 470-1192, Japan

Sekimoto, Mitsugu
Department of Surgery and Clinical Oncology, Graduate School of Medicine, Osaka University
E2, 2-2 Yamadaoka, Suita, Osaka 565-0871, Japan

Shirato, Kunio
Department of Cardiovascular Medicine, Tohoku University Graduate School of Medicine
1-1 Seiryo-machi, Aoba-ku, Sendai 980-8574, Japan

Spöhr, Fabian
Department of Anaesthesiology, University of Heidelberg
Im Neuenheimer Field 110, D-69120 Heidelberg, Germany

Sugimura, Koichiro
Department of Cardiovascular Medicine, Tohoku University Graduate School of Medicine
1-1 Seiryo-machi, Aoba-ku, Sendai 980-8574, Japan

Suzuki, Jun
Department of Cardiovascular Medicine, Tohoku University Graduate School of Medicine
1-1 Seiryo-machi, Aoba-ku, Sendai 980-8574, Japan

Suzuki, Rei
Department of Surgery and Clinical Oncology, Graduate School of Medicine, Osaka University
E2, 2-2 Yamadaoka, Suita, Osaka 565-0871, Japan

Takahashi, Tohru
Department of Cardiovascular Medicine, Tohoku University Graduate School of Medicine
1-1 Seiryo-machi, Aoba-ku, Sendai 980-8574, Japan

Vinciguerra, Giulia
Department of Biomedical Sciences, IRVINE2 Vascular Lab, Chieti University, and San Valentino Vascular Screening Project (Pe)
Via Vespucci 65, 65100 Pescara, Italy

Wang, Huan
Department of Cardiovascular Medicine, Tohoku University Graduate School of Medicine
1-1 Seiryo-machi, Aoba-ku, Sendai 980-8574, Japan

Yamada, Norikazu
First Department of Internal Medicine, Mie University
2-174 Edobashi, Tsu 514-8507, Japan

Yamashita, Mitsuru
Department of Cardiovascular Surgery, Fujita Health University School of Medicine
1-98 Dengakugakubo, Kutsukake-cho, Toyoake, Aichi 470-1192, Japan

1. Epidemiology and Therapy of Acute Pulmonary Thromboembolism

Epidemiology of Pulmonary Embolism in Japan

Masahito Sakuma, Tohru Takahashi, Jun Demachi, Jun Suzuki, Jun Nawata, Noriko Kakudo, Koichiro Sugimura, Boon-Hooi Ong, Huan Wang, Kenya Saji, and Kunio Shirato

Introduction

Pulmonary embolism (PE) is as well recognized a thromboembolic disease, as are cerebral infarction and myocardial infarction in Western countries. However, the number of the patients with PE is still much lower in Japan than in the West. The Ministry of Health, Labor and Welfare in Japan reported in a patient survey that there were 1,220,000 patients with cerebral infarction, 82,000 with myocardial infarction, and only 4,000 with PE in 1999 [1]. Vital statistics in the same year found 51,688 deaths from cerebral infarction, 48,806 from myocardial infarction, and only 1,738 from pulmonary embolism [2]. In this chapter, we show the epidemiological results on PE in Japan, and consider the reasons for the difference in the incidence of PE between Japan and Western countries.

Incidence of Pulmonary Embolism

Vital Statistics

From the point of view of vital statistics, crude deaths from PE rapidly increased, and female deaths exceeded male deaths in the 1990s (Fig. 1) [3]. Age-specific mortality was higher in the elderly and, in recent years, lower in females than in males (Fig. 2) [4]. The results of crude deaths reflect the fact that many more elderly people are female than male. The adjusted mortality in 1996 was 0.71 per 100,000 persons in males and 0.83 in females, which is comparable to the mortality of non-Blacks and non-Whites in the United States [5]. The reduced mortality in the United States was achieved by wide-

Department of Cardiovascular Medicine, Tohoku University Graduate School of Medicine, 1-1 Seiryo-machi, Aoba-ku, Sendai 980-8574, Japan

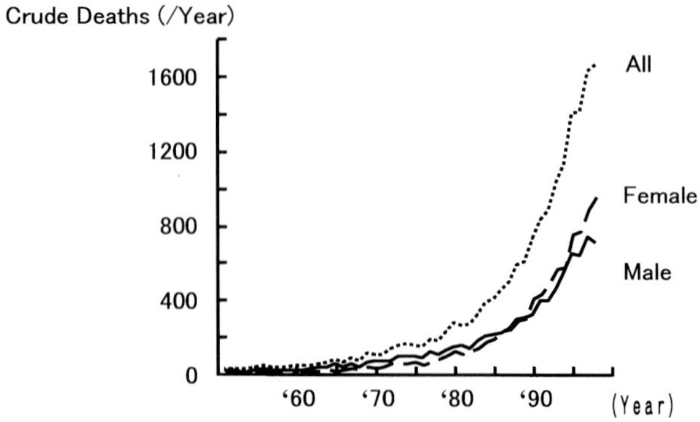

FIG. 1. Crude deaths from pulmonary embolism in Japan. (From [3], with permission)

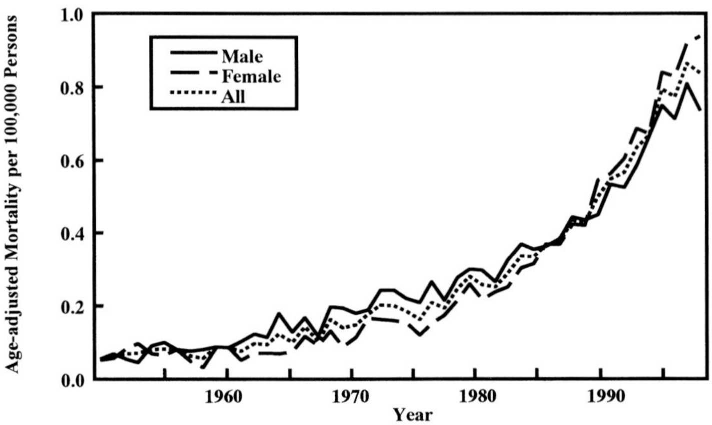

FIG. 2. Age-adjusted mortality from pulmonary embolism in Japan. (From [4], with permission)

spread prevention of venous thromboembolism. Therefore, if prevention is not performed, mortality from PE will further increase in Japan.

Autopsy Studies

Autopsy studies based on data from *Annual of the Pathological Autopsy Cases in Japan* have been analyzed three times [6–8]. Simple comparison among the three studies cannot be done, however, because the entry criteria in these studies were somewhat different. Nevertheless, it is obvious that the rate of PE is increasing in autopsy cases (Fig. 3). The rate of death from PE in many of the autopsy studies ranged from approximately 1% to 5% in Asia and Africa [9–15], which is lower than in Western countries.

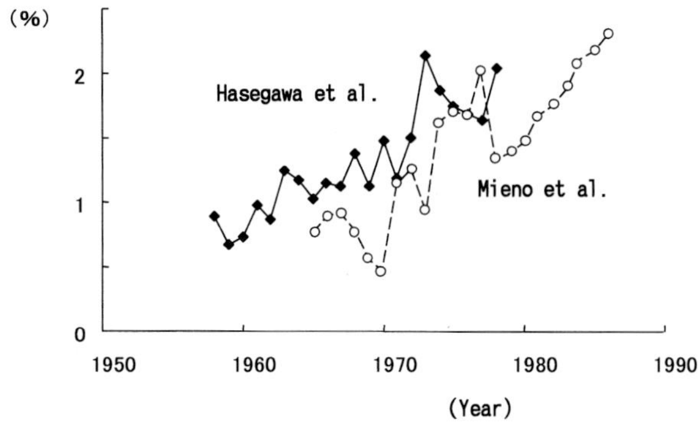

FIG. 3. Rate of cases with pulmonary embolism in autopsy in Japan. (Drawn from the data of [6] and [7])

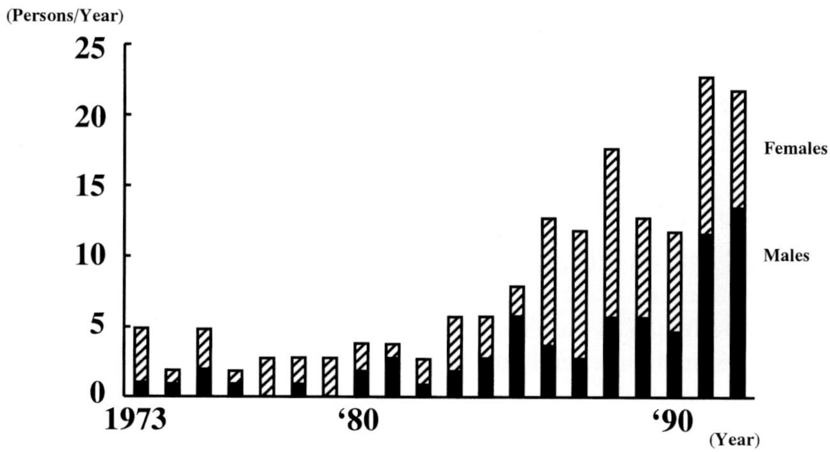

FIG. 4. Pulmonary embolism cases autopsied at Tokyo Medical examiner's office. (From [20], with permission)

In a somewhat older study, the ratio of PE deaths in autopsies was smaller in Japan than in the United States [10]. However, some researchers suggest that the rate is not so low and may be about 20% [16–19]. That is to say, pathologists' recognition of PE may be contributing to the rate of finding PE in autopsies.

Cases of PE increased four to five times from 1973 to 1992 in the Tokyo Medical Examiner's Office (Fig. 4) [20]. The rate of cases with PE was 0.4% during this period. On the other hands, fatal PE in examination cases was 0.9% from 1992 to 2001 in the same institution [21].

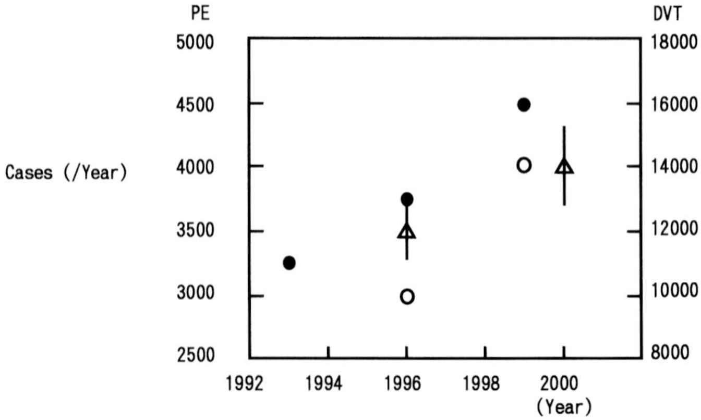

FIG. 5. Clinical cases with pulmonary embolism and venous thrombosis in Japan. △, pulmonary embolism (*PE*) from questionnaire data; ○, PE from patient survey; ●, deep-vein thrombosis (*DVT*) from patient survey. (Drawn from the data of [1], [22–25])

Clinical Surveys

Few clinical data on the incidence or prevalence of PE are available in Japan. Prospective studies using a questionnaire revealed that the incidence of PE was 3,492 patients (28 patients per 1,000,000 people per year) in 1996 [22], and 4,022 (32 patients per 1,000,000 people per year) in 1999 [23] in Japan. The prevalence of PE by patient survey in Japan was 3,000 patients in 1996 [24] and 4,000 in 1999 [1]. These findings indicate that clinical cases with PE increased during the 3 to 4 years. Moreover, the prevalence of deep-vein thrombosis also increased (Fig. 5) [1, 24, 25]. When displaying the ratio of female cases with PE to the 60- to 65-year-old population as a unit, the ratio is higher in females than in males generally, and in elderly people except those 85 years or more of age (Fig. 6) [26].

Silverstein et al. showed that the incidence of PE decreased from the middle 1970s in Olmsted County, Minnesota, USA [27], but clinically diagnosed cases with PE still increased in Japan. Sixty-nine patients per 100,000 people were diagnosed in their report. This ratio is about 20 times higher than that in Japan.

Klatsky et al. [28] examined the relative risks of venous thromboembolism among races. In their report, only Asians had a low relative risk, which was 0.2 (95% confidence interval, 0.1–0.5), when risk among white Americans was construed as 1. This finding shows that, under a fixed diagnostic power, Asians have a low risk for venous thromboembolism compared with Caucasians.

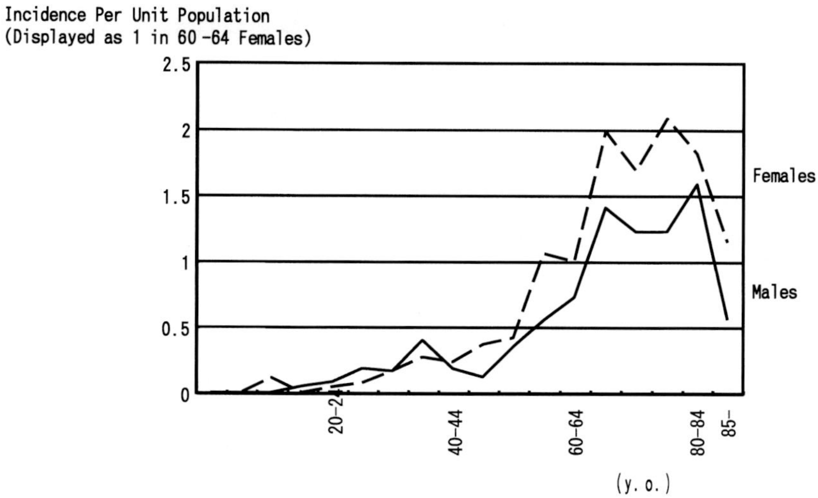

FIG. 6. Distribution of pulmonary embolism by age and by sex in Japan. (Unpublished data)

Clinical Features of Acute Pulmonary Embolism

We describe findings based on the data of the Japanese Society of Pulmonary Embolism Research (JaSPER) in this section. The registry of JaSPER gathered 629 patients with PE including 461 with acute PE, 53 with chronic thromboembolic pulmonary hypertension, 92 with chronic, and 23 with unclassified from November 2000 to August 2003 [29]. A characteristic of PE in Japan is that chronic PE represented a relatively larger part of PE. One of the possible reasons is shown in Okada's report [30]. The patients with chronic thromboembolic pulmonary hypertension have HLA types similar to that in Takayasu's disease, and Takayasu's disease is seen more in Japan than in Western countries. Therefore, he suggested that some inflammation due to a genetic disposition around the pulmonary artery might contribute to the occurrence of chronic pulmonary embolism in Japanese. Outpatients were 58.8% of acute PE. Risk factors of PE in Japan (Fig. 7) were similar to those in previous reports, except in the case of oral contraceptives. In this figure, contraceptives do not appear, because few women use these agents in Japan.

Acute PE was divided into four categories according to the severity of PE at diagnosis. Mortality from PE was 61.5% in cardiopulmonary arrest (52.4% in patients diagnosed before their deaths), 15.6% in shock, 2.7% with right ventricular overload but without shock, and 0.8% without right ventricular overload or shock ($P < 0.0001$) [29].

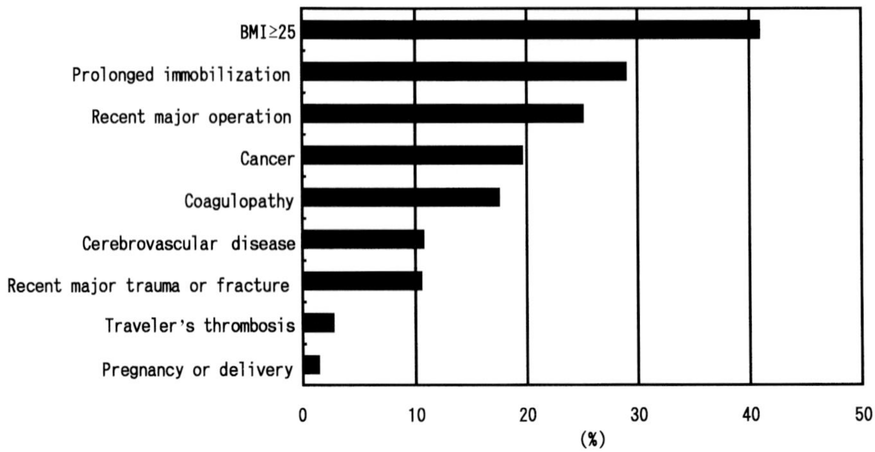

FIG. 7. Risk factors for pulmonary embolism. *BMI*, body mass index. (Unpublished data)

There are two reports on predictors of in-hospital mortality in Japan. Kumasaka et al. [31] indicated that old age (70 years or more), syncope, shock, cerebral infarction, hypocapnia of 25 torr or less, and an elevation of total pulmonary resistance deteriorated the in-hospital outcome (Fig. 8A). Nakamura et al. [32] reported that shock, immobilization, cancer, and male sex worsened the mortality from PE, but thrombolysis did not improve in-hospital deaths (Fig. 8B).

Reasons for Low Incidence and Recent Increment of PE Patients in Japan

There are some reasons why the number of cases with PE are low in Japan compared with that in Western countries. The first is genetic predisposition. Racial differences in congenital coagulopathy have been clarified. The incidence of carriers with factor V Leiden mutation or prothrombin G20210A is high both in the general population and in patients with venous thromboembolism in Western countries [33–36]. However, these mutations have not yet been found in Japanese [37, 38]. The second is lifestyle. In eating habits, Japanese mainly ate rice and beans, relying on fish as animal protein, 30 years ago [39]. Now, we eat less rice and consume more meat than before [39]. Lipid uptake is also increasing. According to the changes in eating habits, the physical constitution in Japanese has changed, for example, body height is gradually increasing. Data are also available about the relationship between obesity and PE. The relation between age and body mass index in the general

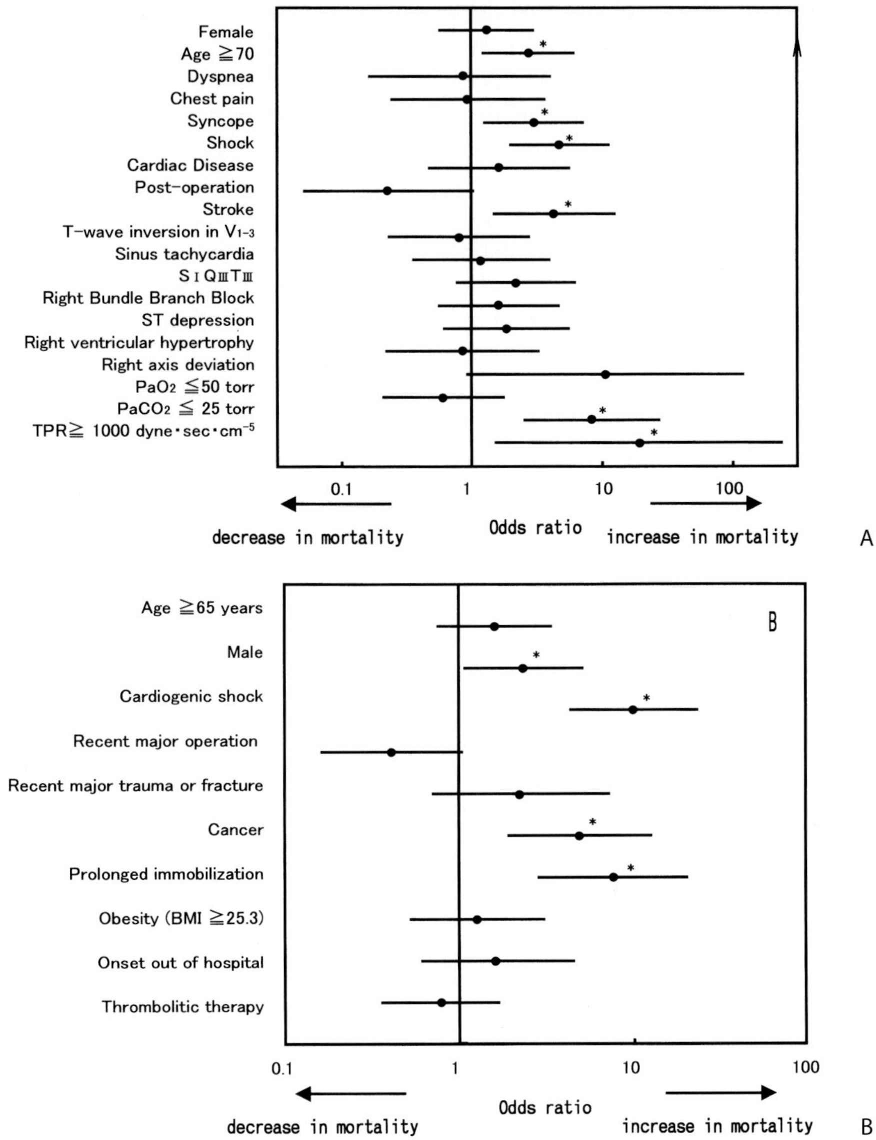

FIG. 8. Predictors of in-hospital mortality in acute pulmonary embolism. *$P < 0.05$. (**A** is drawn from the data of [31]; **B** from the data of [32])

Japanese population from Yoshiike et al. [40] and the data from JaSPER showed that 23 female cases with PE from among 225 exceeded the 95 percentile in the relation between age and body mass index in the general Japanese population ($P = 0.002$), as did 15 male cases from among 137 ($P = 0.03$) (unpublished data). Recently, obesity among males (body mass index 25 or more) has been increasing [41]. However, the number of obese people (body mass index 30 or more) is still low in Japan compared with in Western countries [42]. The third is diagnostic power. In the *Annual of the Pathological Autopsy Cases in Japan*, 13.7% of the patients whose main diagnosis or cause of death was PE at autopsy had been diagnosed as PE clinically in 1987, and this was 26.0% in 1998 [43]. The JaSPER studies showed that less severe cases without shock were 64.1% in the first registry (from January 1994 to October 1997), 69.3% in the second (from November 1997 to October 2000), and 77.7% in the third (November 2000 to August 2003) ($P = 0.0003$) [29, 32, 44]. These findings may indicate that diagnostic power has improved during these 10 years in Japan.

Conclusions

The incidence of PE is low in Japan compared with Western countries, but it has been increasing in recent years. The reasons for the low incidence may be genetic predisposition, lifestyle, and diagnostic power. On the other hand, the recent increment in incidence may result from changes in lifestyle and improvement in the diagnostic power.

References

1. Statistics and Information Department. Patient survey 1999, vol 1. Minister's Secretariat, Ministry of Health, Labor and Welfare, Tokyo, 2001.
2. Statistics and Information Department. Vital statistics of Japan 1999, vol 3. Minister's Secretariat, Ministry of Health, Labor and Welfare, Tokyo, 2001.
3. Sakuma M, Takahashi T, Kitamukai O, et al. Mortality from pulmonary embolism in Japan (in Japanese). J Jpn Coll Angiol 2001;41:2001.
4. Sakuma M, Konno Y, Shirato K. Increasing mortality from pulmonary embolism in Japan, 1951–2000. Circ J 2002;66:1144–9.
5. Lilienfeld DE. Decreasing mortality from pulmonary embolism in the United States, 1979–1996. Int J Epidemiol 2000;29:465–9.
6. Hasegawa H, Nagata H, Yamauchi M, et al. Statistical status of pulmonary embolism in Japan (II). Jpn J Chest Dis 1981;40:677–81 (in Japanese).
7. Mieno T, Kitamura S. Incidence of pulmonary thromboembolism in Japan. Kokyu To Junkan 1989;37:923–7 (in Japanese).
8. Sakuma M, Takahashi T, Kitamukai O, et al. Incidence of pulmonary embolism in Japan: analysis using "Annual of the pathological autopsy cases in Japan." Ther Res 2002;23:632–4 (in Japanese).

9. Thomas WA, Davies JNP, O'Neal RM, et al. Incidence of myocardial infarction correlated with venous and pulmonary thrombosis and embolism: a geographic study based on autopsies in Uganda, East Africa and St. Louis, USA. Am J Cardiol 1960;5:41–7.
10. Gore I, Hirst AE, Tanaka K. Myocardial infarction and thromboembolism. Arch Intern Med 1964;113:323–30.
11. Elegbeleye OO, Femi-Pearse D. Pulmonary embolism in Africans. Trop Geogr Med 1975;27:31–3.
12. Datta BN, Ramesh K, Bhusnurmath B. Autopsy incidence of pulmonary vascular episode: a study of 218 cases. Angiology 1986;37:744–50.
13. Chau KY, Yuen ST, Ng THK, et al. An autopsy study of pulmonary thromboembolism in Hong Kong Chinese. Pathology 1991;23:181–4.
14. Awotedu AA, Igbokwe EO, Akang EE, et al. Pulmonary embolism in Ibadan, Nigeria: five years autopsy report. Cent Afr J Med 1992;38:432–5.
15. Chau KY, Yuen ST, Wong MP. seasonal variation in the necropsy incidence of pulmonary thromboembolism in Hong Kong. J Clin Pathol 1995;48:578–9.
16. Nakano T, Ito S, Takezawa H. Epidemiology of pulmonary embolism. Jpn Med J 1980;2949:43–7 (in Japanese).
17. Matsubara O, Sato T, Kitagawa M, et al. Pulmonary thromboembolism: frequency, site, and vascular change in 103 autopsy cases. Am J Cardiovasc Pathol 1989;2:312–28.
18. Ito M. Pathology of pulmonary embolism. Kokyu To Junkan 1991;39;567–72 (in Japanese).
19. Nakamura Y, Yutani C, Imaike M, et al. Pathophysiology of clinicopathological aspect of venous thrombosis and pulmonary thromboembolism. Jpn J Phlebol 1996;7:17–22 (in Japanese).
20. Murai T. Sudden death due to pulmonary thromboembolism. In: Annual report of the study project of sudden death supported by a Japanese Ministry of Health and Welfare Research Grant 1993, 140–142 (in Japanese).
21. Tanifuji T, Kageyama N, Ro A, et al. A histo-pathological study of fatal pulmonary embolism and deep vein thrombosis: in the study of deep vein thrombosis among forty patients with pulmonary thromboembolism. Jpn J Phlebol 2003;14:189–95 (in Japanese).
22. Kumasaka N, Sakuma M, Shirato K. Incidence of pulmonary thromboembolism in Japan. Jpn Circ J 1999;63:439–41.
23. Kitamukai O, Sakuma M, Takahashi T, et al. Incidence and characteristics of pulmonary thromboembolism in Japan 2000. Intern Med 2003;42:1090–4.
24. Statistics and Information Department. Patient survey 1996, Volume I. Tokyo, 1998.
25. Statistics and Information Department. Patient survey 1993, vol I. Minister's Secretariat, Ministry of Health and Welfare, Tokyo, 1995.
26. The Japanese Society of Pulmonary Embolism Research. Unpublished data.
27. Silverstein MD, Heit JA, Mohr DN, et al. Trends in the incidence of deep vein thrombosis and pulmonary embolism: a 25-year population-based study. Arch Intern Med 1998;158:585–93.
28. Klatsky AL, Armstrong MA, Poggi J. Risk of pulmonary embolism and/or deep venous thrombosis in Asian-Americans. Am J Cardiol 2000;85:1334–7.
29. Sakuma M, Nakamura M, Nakanishi N, et al. The results of the third registry of pulmonary thromboembolism: results of multicenter registry in the Japanese Society of Pulmonary Embolism Research. Ther Res 2004;25:1134–5 (in Japanese).
30. Okada O, Tanebe N, Yasuda J, et al. Comprehensive study for genetic factors in chronic thromboembolic pulmonary hypertension. In: Annual report of the study project of

respiratory failure research committee supported by a Japanese Ministry of Health and Welfare Research Grant 1997. K Planning 1998:140–2 (in Japanese).
31. Kumasaka N, Sakuma M, Shirato K. Clinical features and predictors of in-hospital mortality in patients with acute and chronic pulmonary thromboembolism. Intern Med 2000;39:1038–43.
32. Nakamura M, Fujioka H, Yamada N, et al. Clinical characteristics of acute pulmonary thromboembolism in Japan: results of multicenter registry in the Japanese Society of Pulmonary Embolism Research. Clin Cardiol 2001;24:132–238.
33. Ridker PM, Hennekens CH, Lindpaintner K, et al. Mutation in the gene coding for coagulation factor V and the risk of myocardial infarction, stroke, and venous thrombosis in apparently healthy men. N Engl J Med 1995;332:912–5.
34. Rees DC, Cox M, Clegg JB. World distribution of factor V Leiden. Lancet 1995;346:1133–4.
35. Poort SR, Rosendaal FR, Reitsma PH, et al. A common genetic variation in the 3′-untranslated region of the prothorombin gene is associated with elevated plasma prothrombin levels and an increase in venous thrombosis. Blood 1996;88:3698–703.
36. Tosetto A, Missiaglia E, Frezzato M, et al. The VITA project: prothrombin G20210A mutation and venous thromboembolism in the general population. Thromb Haemostasis 1999;82:1395–8.
37. Seki T, Okayama H, Kumagai T, et al. Arg506Gln mutation of the coagulation factor V gene not detected in Japanese pulmonary thromboembolism. Heart Vessels 1998; 13:195–8.
38. Miyata T, Kawasaki T, Fujimura H, et al. The prothrombin gene G20210A mutation is not found among Japanese patients with deep vein thrombosis and healthy individuals. Blood Coagul Fibrinolysis 1998;9:451–2.
39. The study circle for health and nutrition information. The national nutrition survey in Japan, 2001: Ministry of Health, Labor and Welfare, Japan. Diaachi Shuppan, Tokyo, 2003 (in Japanese).
40. Yoshiike N, Matsumura Y, Zaman MM, et al. Descriptive epidemiology of body mass index in Japanese adults in a representative sample from the National Nutrition Survey 1990–1994. Int J Obes 1998;22:684–7.
41. Tanaka H, Kokubo Y. Epidemiology of obesity. J Jpn Med Assoc 2003;130:25–30 (in Japanese).
42. WHO. Obesity: preventing and managing the global epidemic. Report of a WHO consultation. WHO technical report series, no 894. World Health Organization, Geneva, 2000.
43. Sakuma M, Takahashi T, Kitamukai O, et al. Autopsy incidence of pulmonary thromboembolism. Ther Res 2002;23:632–4 (in Japanese).
44. Sakuma M, Okada O, Nakamura M, et al. Recent developments in diagnostic imaging techniques and management for acute pulmonary embolism: multicenter registry by the Japanese Society of pulmonary Embolism research. Intern Med 2003;42:470–6.

Thrombolytic Treatment of Acute Pulmonary Embolism: Toward the End of a Long-Lasting Debate?

Stavros Konstantinides

More than 30 years have passed since the first reports on the use of thrombolytic agents in acute pulmonary embolism (PE). During this time, experimental studies, clinical observations, and randomized trials consistently demonstrated the favorable effects of thrombolysis on angiographic, hemodynamic, and scintigraphic parameters of patients with acute PE. However, this evidence has not been translated into a wide clinical acceptance of thrombolytic agents by the clinicians caring for patients with acute PE. In particular, there is an ongoing "thrombolysis debate" regarding the appropriate treatment of patients with *submassive* PE. These patients present with evidence of right ventricular dysfunction, particularly echocardiographic signs of right ventricular enlargement and/or hypokinesis, but have no hemodynamic instability such as persistent hypotension or shock at diagnosis.

The arguments of the investigators opposing the use of thrombolysis in pulmonary embolism can be summarized in the following points [1, 2]: (1) with the exception of massive PE resulting in cardiogenic shock, thrombolytic therapy of PE does not reduce in-hospital or long-term mortality compared to heparin alone; (2) the hemodynamic benefits of thrombolytic agents are confined to the first few days (or hours) after the beginning of treatment; and (3) thrombolysis is potentially life-threatening treatment due to its high bleeding risk. In fact, the existing data from the few randomized thrombolysis trials performed to date appear to support these conclusions at first sight. However, when carefully examined in their context, the results of the studies on PE management and prognosis actually support the use of thrombolysis in addition to heparin anticoagulation in patients with submassive PE.

As early as 1971, Miller et al. showed that streptokinase infusion over 72 h resulted in a significant reduction of systolic pulmonary artery pressure, total

---

Department of Cardiology and Pulmonary Medicine, Georg August University, Robert Koch Strasse 40, D-37075 Goettingen, Germany; E-mail: skonstan@med.uni-goettingen.de

pulmonary resistance, and the angiographic index of PE severity [3]. In comparison, conventional heparin anticoagulation had no appreciable effect on the these parameters during the first 3 days. During the following 30 years, the angiographic and hemodynamic benefits of thrombolysis were confirmed in nine controlled randomized trials that compared various regimens of streptokinase, urokinase, or recombinant tissue plasminogen activator (alteplase) with heparin alone in the treatment of acute PE (Table 1).

The results of these series, most of which included only few (between 8 and 53) patients, were recently reviewed in two meta-analyses with almost identical results [4, 5]. Of note, however, only two of the nine trials were large enough to include more than 100 patients. The first one, the Urokinase Pulmonary Embolism Trial (UPET), enrolled 160 patients and was, until a few months ago, the largest randomized thrombolysis trial in patients with pulmonary embolism. In UPET, administration of urokinase (4,400 U/kg bolus injection followed by an infusion of 4,400 U/kg/h over 24 h) was superior to heparin alone in resolving pulmonary artery thrombi [6]. In some patients, this effect appeared to result in clinical stabilization and reversal of the signs of cardiogenic shock. However, during the 2-week follow-up period, overall mortality was not significantly affected by thrombolytic treatment (7.3% in the urokinase versus 9.0% in the heparin group), and the incidence of recurrent PE also was not reduced (17.1% vs. 23.1%). Because of its size and the seemingly disappointing results, UPET has frequently been cited as the "proof" that thrombolysis is not indicated in acute PE. However, when interpreting these data and discussing their implications for clinical practice, it is important to keep in mind that UPET and all the other thrombolysis trials conducted between 1973 and 1993 insisted on angiographic confirmation of PE for patient inclusion, and defined the severity of PE on the basis of angiographic or scintigraphic rather than clinical criteria (see Table 1). Furthermore, these studies focused on hemodynamic and angiographic rather than clinical endpoints to determine the efficacy of thrombolytic treatment (Table 1). At that time, following these rigid methodological principles was thought to guarantee the quality of the data and permit objective comparisons between therapeutic regimens. On the other hand, these design characteristics also meant that the majority of the thrombolysis trials in PE could not identify the appropriate candidates for thrombolytic treatment and did not address the benefits of thrombolysis with regard to the patients' outcome. In fact, it is even possible some of the trials inadvertently "selected" patients who were stable enough to be transported from the emergency room or the intensive care unit to undergo time-consuming angiographic or scintigraphic procedures before enrollment. This somewhat provocative thesis is supported by the Management Strategy and Prognosis of Pulmonary Embolism Registry (MAPPET), which found that patients with confirmation of PE by pulmonary

TABLE 1. Thrombolytic treatment versus heparin alone in acute pulmonary embolism: prospective randomized studies over a 30-year period

Study/author	Year	Patients (*n*)	Treatment groups (*n*)	Inclusion criteria		Follow-up (days)	Primary endpoint
				PE diagnosis	PE severity		
UPET [6]	1973	160	UK (82) Heparin (78)	Angiography, LS	—	14	Angiographic (reperfusion), hemodynamic (PAP)
Tibbutt [36]	1974	30	SK i.p. (13) Heparin (17)	Angiography	Massive PE	3	Angiographic (reperfusion)
Ly [37]	1978	25	SK (14) Heparin (11)	Angiography	>1 lobar artery	10	Angiographic (reperfusion)
Marini [38]	1988	30	UK (20) Heparin (10)	Angiography, LS	>9 nonperfused segments	7	LS (reperfusion)
PIOPED [39]	1990	13	rtPA (9) Heparin (4)	Angiography, LS	>1 lobar *or* >2 segmental arteries	7	Hemodynamic (PAP)
Levine [15]	1990	58	rtPA (33) Heparin (25)	Angiography, LS	—	10	LS (reperfusion)
PAIMS-2 [12]	1992	36	rtPA (20) Heparin (16)	Angiography	Miller score >11	7	Angiographic (reperfusion), hemodynamic (PAP)
Goldhaber [8]	1993	101	rtPA (46) Heparin (55)	Angiography, LS, echo	—	14	Echocardiographic (RV function)
Jerjes-Sanchez [9][a]	1995	8	SK (4) Heparin (4)	Angiography	>9 nonperfused segments, *or* <9 segments plus RV dysfunction	3	LS (reperfusion)
MAPPET-3 [19]	2002	256	rtPA (118) Heparin (138)	Echo, LS, CT	RV dysfunction	30	Clinical (mortality, complications)

CT, (spiral) computer tomography; i.p., intrapulmonary administration; echo, echocardiography; LS, lung scan; MAPPET, Management Strategy and Prognosis of Pulmonary Embolism Study; *n*, number of patients included in each study, or number of patients in each treatment group; PAIMS, Plasminogen Activator Italian Multicenter Study; PAP, pulmonary artery pressure; PE, pulmonary embolism; PIOPED, Prospective Investigation of Pulmonary Embolism Diagnosis; RV, right ventricular; rtPA, recombinant tissue plasminogen activator; SK, streptokinase; UK, urokinase; UPET, Urokinase Pulmonary Embolism Trial

[a] This study was terminated prematurely due to the extremely poor outcome in the heparin-only group

angiography or lung scan had a much lower death rate than those in whom the diagnosis was based on clinical, ECG, and echocardiographic findings alone [7]. It is, indeed, not hard to imagine that the extent and invasiveness of the diagnostic workup for suspected PE can be influenced by the severity of clinical instability at presentation.

The only major thrombolysis trial besides UPET was published by Goldhaber et al. in 1993 and compared alteplase (100 mg infusion over 2 h) to heparin alone [8]. This trial included 101 patients and was the first to apply echocardiographic indicators of right ventricular pressure overload and dysfunction in the evaluation of PE severity. The authors reported that pathognomonic ultrasound findings were present in 54% of the patients included, but the study did not exclude patients with a normally functioning right ventricle on echocardiography. Thus, the study included but did not focus on the patient population with submassive PE. An important finding of Goldhaber's trial was the rapid improvement of right ventricular function in the alteplase group as assessed by 24-hour echocardiographic follow-up. However, thrombolysis was again not shown to have any effect on survival, partly because of the low (2%) overall in-hospital mortality. Therefore, the opponents of thrombolysis are obviously right when they state that, with the exception of massive PE resulting in cardiogenic shock [9], thrombolytic therapy of PE has not been shown to reduce in-hospital or long-term mortality compared to heparin alone [4, 5].

Thrombolysis undoubtedly results in rapid (within a few hours) resolution of pulmonary emboli and thus in normalization of the pressures in the pulmonary circulation and right ventricle. However, early studies showed that "spontaneous" resolution of PE also occurs in patients treated with heparin alone, although it may take considerably longer (2 to 3 weeks) [10]. In a prospective hemodynamic and echocardiographic study, our group compared the effects of alteplase treatment with those of heparin alone in 40 patients with acute submassive and massive PE [11]. Significant reduction of pulmonary artery pressure and total pulmonary resistance together with an increase in cardiac output was observed within the first 12 h in the alteplase (but not in the heparin) group, thus confirming previous observations [12, 13]. Furthermore, patients treated with alteplase had rapid normalization of the diameter of the right and the left ventricle as assessed by echocardiography. By the end of the first week, however, no difference existed between the two treatment groups regarding the overall change in right or left heart chamber dimensions, or the incidence of right ventricular dilation and paradoxical septal wall motion. Thus, it cannot be disputed that the benefits of thrombolysis (when compared with heparin alone) in the treatment of PE are, indeed, short lived, as stated by the opponents of thrombolysis. The critical issue in this regard is whether the rapid normalization of hemodynamic parameters can affect the prognosis of (some) patients substantially enough to justify the potential risks of thrombolytic agents.

The risk of life-threatening or disabling hemorrhage associated with thrombolysis is undoubtedly a reason for concern. Pooling the data from all major thrombolysis trials conducted since 1973 [6, 12, 14–19], including those studies designed to compare different thrombolytic regimens, a 19% rate of major bleeding complications and a 2% rate of intracranial and/or fatal hemorrhage can be calculated (Table 2). On the other hand, if the data from retrospective cohort studies and registries [20–23] are used as a source, the incidence of major bleeding events is as high as 36% and that of intracranial/fatal hemorrhage amounts to 4% (Table 2). It is possible that complication rates are so much higher in registries because the clinicians decided in some cases that the patient's situation justified use of thrombolytic agents despite the presence of formal contraindications. However, there can be little doubt that thrombolytic agents are potentially dangerous drugs and should be reserved for high-risk patients whose condition requires rapid resolution of the emboli in the pulmonary circulation. It is thus the clinician's task to identify and select those high-risk patients in whom thrombolysis is warranted. For example, massive PE with cardiogenic shock is widely accepted as a life-threatening situation demanding immediate thrombolysis. However, the prognosis of patients with submassive PE may also be poor enough to justify "aggressive" treatment, as is discussed next.

Because the opponents of thrombolysis in PE are right in all their arguments [1, 2], as already explained, thrombolytic agents are not acceptable as standard treatment of unselected patients with acute PE. How is it then possible to select the high-risk patients for whom thrombolysis may have a favorable risk-to-benefit ratio?

The existing data on the clinical course and prognosis of acute PE appear "controversial" at first sight. Massive PE presenting with clinical instability is undoubtedly a life-threatening situation, as 18% of patients with massive PE died in the series of Hall et al. [24], and death rates approached or exceeded 30% in other reports on patients presenting with cardiogenic shock due to right heart failure [25, 26]. On the other hand, 1-year mortality was reported to be as low as 1% in a multicenter study performed by the British Thoracic Society to determine the optimal duration of anticoagulation for unselected patients with venous thromboembolism [27]. These apparently conflicting reports indicate that patients with acute PE comprise a heterogeneous population whose prognosis and clinical course should be stratified rather than globally determined.

Dysfunction and failure of the right ventricle is now recognized as the crucial event in the pathophysiology of acute PE [28]. For example, the presence of acute right ventricular dilatation on echocardiography was reported

TABLE 2. Bleeding complications of thrombolytic treatment in patients with acute pulmonary embolism

Study/author/year	Study design	Thrombolytic agent	Bleeding rates in the thrombolysis group	
			Major bleeding (n/N)	Intracranial or fatal bleeding (n/N)
UPET 1973 [6]	Prospective, randomized	UK vs. heparin	37/82	1/82
USPET 1974 [14]	Prospective, randomized	UK vs. SK (no heparin group)	32/113	0/113
			12/54	0/54
Levine 1990 [15]	Prospective, randomized	rtPA vs. heparin	0/33	0/33
PAIMS-2 1992 [12]	Prospective, randomized	rtPA vs. heparin	4/20	2/20
Meyer 1992 [16]	Prospective, randomized	rtPA vs. UK (no heparin group)	7/34	1/34
			8/29	1/29
Sors 1994 [17]	Prospective, randomized	Two regimens of rtPA (no heparin group)	0/53	0/53
Kanter and Goldhaber 1997 [18]	Meta-analysis (5 prospective studies) [8, 13, 40–42]	rtPA vs. UK (or vs. heparin)	—	6/312
MAPPET-3 2002 [19]	Prospective, randomized	rtPA vs. heparin	1/118	0/118
Overall (prospective thrombolysis studies)			101/536 (19%)	11/536 (2.0%)
MAPPET 1997 [23]	Registry (prospective)	Various	37/169	2/169
Meyer 1998 [22]	Retrospective	rtPA	33/132	2/132
ICOPER 1999 [21]	Registry (prospective)	Various	66/304	9/304
Hamel 2001 [20]	Registry (retrospective)	Various	6/64	3/64
Overall (registries/ retrospective studies)			142/399 (36%)	16/399 (4.0%)

ICOPER, International Cooperative Pulmonary Embolism Registry; MAPPET, Management Strategy and Prognosis of Pulmonary Embolism Registry; n, number of patients with major or intracranial/fatal bleeding, respectively, in each study; N, number of patients treated with a thrombolytic agent in each study; PAIMS, Plasminogen Activator Italian Multicenter Study; rtPA, recombinant tissue plasminogen activator; SK, streptokinase; UK, urokinase; UPET, Urokinase Pulmonary Embolism Trial; USPET, Urokinase-Streptokinase Pulmonary Embolism Trial

to be associated with increased in-hospital mortality in patients presenting with suspected PE [29]. In fact, two large multicenter registries [7, 21] and a prospective cohort study [30] confirmed that clinical, hemodynamic, and echocardiographic findings indicating overt *or impending* right heart failure (i.e., massive or submassive PE) independently predict an adverse outcome (mortality rate, 8% or higher) during the hospital stay. In comparison, the risk of death from acute PE is less than 1% in the absence of such findings [29, 30]. More recently, a number of studies consistently demonstrated that elevated cardiac troponin I or T levels may also be a reliable indicator of damage to the right ventricular myocardium and a poor prognosis in patients with PE [31–33]. These laboratory markers can thus become a useful alternative to echocardiography in identifying high-risk patients with PE.

Based on these considerations, it seems reasonable to assume that patients with right ventricular dysfunction may be those who will benefit from thrombolytic treatment. In fact, apart from identifying predictors of outcome in acute PE, the Management Strategies and Prognosis of Pulmonary Embolism (MAPPET) registry also found that early thrombolytic treatment of clinically stable patients with echocardiographic evidence of impending right heart failure was associated with an almost 50% reduction in the risk of in-hospital death [23]. Although this was not a randomized trial, its findings in a large patient population provided a first link between the hemodynamic benefits of thrombolysis and (possibly) a favorable impact on the prognosis of patients with submassive PE.

The promising observations from the MAPPET registry provided the background for the recently published MAPPET-3 Study, the largest prospective randomized thrombolysis trial to date [19]. Patients included in MAPPET-3 had acute submassive PE with evidence of pulmonary hypertension or right ventricular dysfunction. The 256 patients enrolled were randomly asigned to receive alteplase or placebo with concomitant heparin anticoagulation. The primary endpoint of the study was in-hospital death or need for escalation of treatment, defined as catecholamine administration, emergency thrombolysis, endotracheal intubation, cardiopulmonary resuscitation, or emergency surgical embolectomy or catheter thrombus fragmentation. Alteplase treatment reduced the incidence of the primary endpoint from 25% to 11%, a highly significant difference. Although in-hospital mortality was not significantly different between the alteplase and the heparin-only group (see Table 1), this study showed for the first time that early treatment with alteplase can improve the *clinical* course of patients with acute submassive PE, and particularly that it can reduce the risk of clinical deterioration requiring emergency thrombolysis [34]. Importantly, no fatal or cerebral bleeding episodes were observed in the alteplase group (see Table 2). This fact indicates that thrombolysis can be safe in patients who have no contraindications to this type of treatment.

At present, it is uncertain whether further large thrombolysis trials will be conducted in the future and if they will show a survival benefit for patients with submassive PE. On the other hand, it needs to be emphasized that composite endpoints assessing both mortality and major complications (requiring emergency treatment) have become the standard means of assessing patient outcome in major therapeutic trials; this is partly due to ethical considerations, which require that everything be done to protect the lives of the patients enrolled. In fact, the results of MAPPET-3 suggest that prompt escalation of therapy in response to clinical or hemodynamic deterioration could rescue many lives even in the group initially treated with heparin alone.

In conclusion, it can be stated at present that we have found the answers to some of the critical questions concerning the management of PE. In particular, evidence has recently accumulated that patients with acute submassive PE have a mortality risk that is high enough to require more aggressive treatment than heparin alone. As an alternative to echocardiography, when this diagnostic modality is not available or yields nonconclusive results, simple laboratory tools such as the cardiac troponins I and T, and possibly the pro-brain natriuretic peptide (BNP) levels as well [35], have been developed for identifying high-risk patients, and they have already been shown to predict the outcome of patients with confirmed PE. Based on these considerations, if echocardiography reveals the presence of right ventricular dysfunction, and particularly if cardiac troponin I or T levels in serum are also elevated, the diagnosis of submassive (or massive) PE can be made. Treatment should be instituted promptly or heparin anticoagulation continued, if already started. On the basis of the MAPPET-3 data, thrombolytic treatment should strongly be considered, even if blood pressure is (still) normal. On the other hand, if it is initially decided to proceed with "watchful waiting" in a patient with submassive PE, close monitoring in the ICU is mandatory and emergency thrombolysis is warranted as soon as the patient's condition appears to deteriorate.

References

1. Dalen JE, Alpert JS, Hirsch J. Thrombolytic therapy for pulmonary embolism: is it effective? Is it safe? When is it indicated? Arch Intern Med 1997;157:2550–6.
2. Dalen JE. The uncertain role of thrombolytic therapy in the treatment of pulmonary embolism. Arch Intern Med 2002;162:2521–3.
3. Miller GA, Sutton GC, Kerr IH, et al. Comparison of streptokinase and heparin in treatment of isolated acute massive pulmonary embolism. Br Heart J 1971;33:616.
4. Agnelli G, Becattini C, Kirschstein T. Thrombolysis vs. heparin in the treatment of pulmonary embolism: a clinical outcome-based meta-analysis. Arch Intern Med 2002;162:2537–41.
5. Thabut G, Thabut D, Myers RP, et al. Thrombolytic therapy of pulmonary embolism: a meta-analysis. J Am Coll Cardiol 2002;40:1660–7.

6. The urokinase pulmonary embolism trial. A national cooperative study. Circulation 1973;47:II1–108.
7. Kasper W, Konstantinides S, Geibel A, et al. Management strategies and determinants of outcome in acute major pulmonary embolism: results of a multicenter registry. J Am Coll Cardiol 1997;30:1165–71.
8. Goldhaber SZ, Haire WD, Feldstein ML, et al. Alteplase versus heparin in acute pulmonary embolism: randomised trial assessing right-ventricular function and pulmonary perfusion. Lancet 1993;341:507–11.
9. Jerjes-Sanchez C, Ramírez-Rivera A, de Lourdes G, et al. Streptokinase and heparin versus heparin alone in massive pulmonary embolism: a randomized controlled trial. J Thromb Thrombolysis 1995;2:227–9.
10. Dalen JE, Banas JS Jr, Brooks HL, et al. Resolution rate of acute pulmonary embolism in man. N Engl J Med 1969;280:1194–9.
11. Konstantinides S, Tiede N, Geibel A, et al. Comparison of alteplase versus heparin for resolution of major pulmonary embolism. Am J Cardiol 1998;82:966–70.
12. Dalla-Volta S, Palla A, Santolicandro A, et al. PAIMS 2: alteplase combined with heparin versus heparin in the treatment of acute pulmonary embolism. Plasminogen activator Italian multicenter study 2. J Am Coll Cardiol 1992;20:520–6.
13. Goldhaber SZ, Vaughan DE, Markis JE, et al. Acute pulmonary embolism treated with tissue plasminogen activator. Lancet 1986;2:886–9.
14. Urokinase-streptokinase embolism trial. Phase 2 results. A cooperative study. JAMA 1974;229:1606–13.
15. Levine M, Hirsh J, Weitz J, et al. A randomized trial of a single bolus dosage regimen of recombinant tissue plasminogen activator in patients with acute pulmonary embolism. Chest 1990;98:1473–9.
16. Meyer G, Sors H, Charbonnier B, et al. Effects of intravenous urokinase versus alteplase on total pulmonary resistance in acute massive pulmonary embolism: a European multicenter double-blind trial. The European Cooperative Study Group for Pulmonary Embolism [see comments]. J Am Coll Cardiol 1992;19:239–45.
17. Sors H, Pacouret G, Azarian R, et al. Hemodynamic effects of bolus vs. 2-h infusion of alteplase in acute massive pulmonary embolism. A randomized controlled multicenter trial. Chest 1994;106:712–17.
18. Kanter DS, Mikkola KM, Patel SR, et al. Thrombolytic therapy for pulmonary embolism. Frequency of intracranial hemorrhage and associated risk factors [comment]. Chest 1997;111:1241–5.
19. Konstantinides S, Geibel A, Heusel G, et al. Heparin plus alteplase compared with heparin alone in patients with submassive pulmonary embolism. N Engl J Med 2002;347:1143–50.
20. Hamel E, Pacouret G, Vincentelli D, et al. Thrombolysis or heparin therapy in massive pulmonary embolism with right ventricular dilation: results from a 128-patient monocenter registry. Chest 2001;120:120–5.
21. Goldhaber SZ, Visani L, De Rosa M. Acute pulmonary embolism: clinical outcomes in the International Cooperative Pulmonary Embolism Registry (ICOPER). Lancet 1999;353:1386–9.
22. Meyer G, Gisselbrecht M, Diehl JL, et al. Incidence and predictors of major hemorrhagic complications from thrombolytic therapy in patients with massive pulmonary embolism. Am J Med 1998;105:472–7.
23. Konstantinides S, Geibel A, Olschewski M, et al. Association between thrombolytic treatment and the prognosis of hemodynamically stable patients with major pulmonary embolism: results of a multicenter registry. Circulation 1997;96:882–8.
24. Hall RJ, Sutton GC, Kerr IH. Long-term prognosis of treated acute massive pulmonary embolism. Br Heart J 1977;39:1128–34.

25. Gulba DC, Schmid C, Borst HG, et al. Medical compared with surgical treatment for massive pulmonary embolism. Lancet 1994;343:576–7.
26. Alpert JS, Smith R, Carlson J, et al. Mortality in patients treated for pulmonary embolism. JAMA 1976;236:1477–80.
27. Optimum duration of anticoagulation for deep-vein thrombosis and pulmonary embolism. Research Committee of the British Thoracic Society. Lancet 1992;340:873–6.
28. Lualdi JC, Goldhaber SZ. Right ventricular dysfunction after acute pulmonary embolism: pathophysiologic factors, detection, and therapeutic implications. Am Heart J 1995;130:1276–82.
29. Kasper W, Konstantinides S, Geibel A, et al. Prognostic significance of right ventricular afterload stress detected by echocardiography in patients with clinically suspected pulmonary embolism. Heart 1997;77:346–9.
30. Grifoni S, Olivotto I, Cecchini P, et al. Short-term clinical outcome of patients with acute pulmonary embolism, normal blood pressure, and echocardiographic right ventricular dysfunction. Circulation 2000;101:2817–22.
31. Janata K, Holzer M, Laggner AN, et al. Cardiac troponin T in the severity assessment of patients with pulmonary embolism: cohort study. BMJ 2003;326:312–13.
32. Konstantinides S, Geibel A, Olschewski M, et al. Importance of cardiac troponins I and T in risk stratification of patients with acute pulmonary embolism. Circulation 2002;106:1263–8.
33. Giannitsis E, Muller-Bardorff M, Kurowski V, et al. Independent prognostic value of cardiac troponin T in patients with confirmed pulmonary embolism. Circulation 2000;102:211–17.
34. Goldhaber SZ. Thrombolysis for pulmonary embolism. N Engl J Med 2002;347:1131–2.
35. Kucher N, Printzen G, Doernhoefer T, et al. Low pro-brain natriuretic peptide levels predict benign clinical outcome in acute pulmonary embolism. Circulation 2003;107:1576–8.
36. Tibbutt DA, Davies JA, Anderson JA, et al. Comparison by controlled clinical trial of streptokinase and heparin in treatment of life-threatening pulmonay embolism. Br Med J 1974;1:343–7.
37. Ly B, Arnesen H, Eie H, et al. A controlled clinical trial of streptokinase and heparin in the treatment of major pulmonary embolism. Acta Med Scand 1978;203:465–70.
38. Marini C, Di Ricco G, Rossi G, et al. Fibrinolytic effects of urokinase and heparin in acute pulmonary embolism: a randomized clinical trial. Respiration 1988;54:162–73.
39. Tissue plasminogen activator for the treatment of acute pulmonary embolism. A collaborative study by the PIOPED Investigators. Chest 1990;97:528–33.
40. Goldhaber SZ, Agnelli G, Levine MN. Reduced dose bolus alteplase vs. conventional alteplase infusion for pulmonary embolism thrombolysis. An international multicenter randomized trial. The Bolus Alteplase Pulmonary Embolism Group. Chest 1994;106:718–24.
41. Goldhaber SZ, Kessler CM, Heit JA, et al. Recombinant tissue-type plasminogen activator versus a novel dosing regimen of urokinase in acute pulmonary embolism: a randomized controlled multicenter trial. J Am Coll Cardiol 1992;20:24–30.
42. Goldhaber SZ, Kessler CM, Heit J, et al. Randomised controlled trial of recombinant tissue plasminogen activator versus urokinase in the treatment of acute pulmonary embolism. Lancet 1988;2:293–8.

The Efficacy of Pharmacomechanical Thrombolysis in the Treatment of Acute Pulmonary Thromboembolism and Deep Venous Thrombosis

N. Yamada

Introduction

Various new intravascular techniques are being tested in the treatment of deep venous thrombosis (DVT) and acute pulmonary thromboembolism (APTE). Among the thrombolytic methods of treating DVT, catheter-directed thrombolysis that administers medication locally to the thrombus has shown a superior, early thrombolytic effect compared to conventional peripheral vein administration [1–4]. However, with regard to thrombolytic treatment of APTE, no significant difference in therapeutic effect has so far been shown between administration in the pulmonary artery using a catheter and systemic administration from a peripheral vein [5]. We therefore studied pharmacomechanical thrombolysis (PMT) by the pulse spray method, which differs from the conventional infusion method by forcefully spraying fluid from multiple holes in a catheter placed at the thrombus site, thereby mechanically macerating the thrombus. Preliminary data of PMT use in massive or submassive APTE and therapeutic effect in acute stage proximal DVT are reported here.

Subjects and Methods

Study 1

The subjects were seven cases of massive or submassive APTE (three men, four women; average age, 57.7 ± 15.0 years). Cases contraindicated for thrombolytic therapy and patients more than 80 years of age were excluded from the study. Subjects were divided into two groups, one group of systemic

First Department of Internal Medicine, Mie University, 2-174 Edobashi, Tsu 514-8507, Japan

administration of a thrombolytic agent from a peripheral vein (group S) and a PMT group (group P), and the therapeutic effect and complications were compared between the two groups. The thrombolytic agent used was monteplase; the dose was 27,500 units/kg administered for about 2 min. When we could confirm pretreatment proximal DVT by venous ultrasonography of the lower extremities or ascending venography, or if we did not have sufficient time to find the source of the embolism, the patients were given thrombolysis after implantation of a non-permanent inferior vena cava filter. In the PMT group, we inserted a guidewire into the region where the largest thrombi were identified by pulmonary arteriography, then used the Fountain infusion system (Merit Medical). The monteplase solution was diluted by normal saline and forcefully sprayed on the thrombi through the catheter several times, 1 ml at a time, for about 2 min. Right heart catheterization and pulmonary arteriography were conducted before and 1 h after PMT, and treatment results were evaluated. The modified Miller index was used to assess thrombus volume observed by pulmonary arteriography. For the left or right pulmonary artery with a greater degree of occlusion as shown by pretreatment pulmonary arteriography, assessment was carried out as shown in Fig. 1. Each part of the pulmonary artery was given a number based on the extent of intravascular thrombi (3, total occlusion; 2, more than half of the lumen occluded; 1, less than half of the lumen occluded), and the numbers were mul-

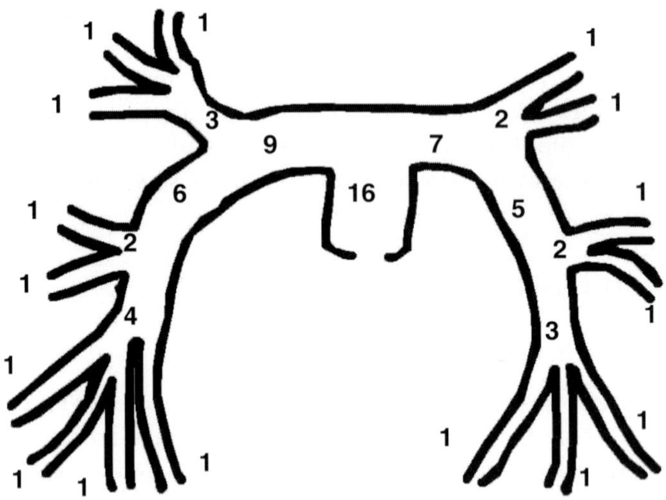

Fig. 1. Modified Miller index. The extent of thrombus in each part of the pulmonary arteries was assessed as follows: total occlusion (3 points), more than half of the part (2 points), less than half (1 point), or none (0). The index score is these points multiplied by the score of each part of the pulmonary arteries

TABLE 1. Venographic severity score

Segment	Score
Inferior vena cava: upper	0 No thrombus
Inferior vena cava: middle	1 Thrombus extended over 1/3 of the length of venous segment without occlusion
Inferior vena cava: lower	2 Thrombus extended over 2/3 of the length of venous segment without occlusion
Common iliac vein	3 Thrombus extended to entire length of venous segment without occlusion
External iliac vein	4 Thrombus extended over 1/3 of the length of venous segment with occlusion
Common femoral vein	5 Thrombus extended over 2/3 of the length of venous segment with occlusion
Superficial femoral vein: proximal	6 Thrombus extended to entire length of venous segment with occlusion
Superficial femoral vein: distal	
Popliteal vein	

tiplied by the score of each part of the pulmonary arteries to obtain an index score.

Study 2

The subjects were 23 cases of acute proximal DVT (11 men, 12 women; average age, 54.5 ± 14.3 years) who were administered PMT. Using the venographic severity (VS) scores (Table 1) based on pre- and post-PMT venography, scores of the evaluated regions were tallied to assess the acute-stage thrombolytic effect. To prevent APTE that occurs during treatment, non-permanent inferior vena cava filters were implanted pre-PMT in all patients. A guidewire was passed through the occluded region and the catheter was positioned so that the medication would be sprayed directly on the thrombi. In all cases the catheter was inserted in an orthodromic direction to avoid injury to the venous valve. The non-permanent inferior vena cava filter was removed post-PMT after confirming by cavography or contrast-enhanced computed tomography (CT) that no thrombi were trapped in the filter.

Furthermore, studies 1 and 2 used unfractionated heparin as the anticoagulant and adjusted the dose so that the APTT (activated partial thromboplastin time) would be 2.0–2.5 times the control.

Results

Study 1

After allocating the patients to two groups, there were three in group S and four in group P. Patient backgrounds were as follows (group S versus group P): average age, 55.3 ± 11.1 years versus 59.5 ± 19.0 years, no shock at onset

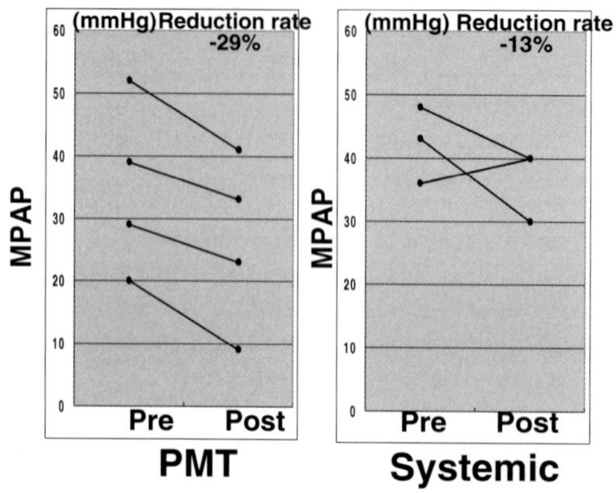

FIG. 2. Improvement rate of mean pulmonary arterial pressure between pretreatment and posttreatment. *Left*, P group; *right*, S group; *MPAP*, mean pulmonary arterial pressure; *PMT*, pharmacomechanical thrombolysis

TABLE 2. Improvement rate between pretreatment and posttreatment modified Miller index

	PMT ($n = 4$)	Systemic ($n = 3$)
Pre	46.5 ± 29.2	23.3 ± 16.0
Post	17.8 ± 13.9	11.0 ± 14.2
Improvement rate	61.7%	52.8%

PMT, pharmacomechanical thrombolysis

in either group, two versus two syncope cases, and echocardiography findings revealing right heart overload in all cases. Inferior vena cava filters were used in a total of four cases, three with the Günther tulip filter (manufactured by Cook) and one with the Antheor filter (manufactured by Boston Scientific). The improvement rate of the mean arterial pressure (pre-PMT–post-PMT/pre-PMT levels) was 13% in group S and higher, 29%, in group P (Fig. 2), and the modified Miller index used as an indicator of thrombolysis on the pulmonary arteriogram was 23.3 ± 16.0 to 11.0 ± 14.2, an improvement rate of 52.8%, in group S, and 46.5 ± 29.2 to 17.8 ± 13.9, an improvement rate of 61.7%, in group P. There was no statistically significant difference- because of the limited number of patients, but group P had a higher rate (Table 2, Fig. 3). With regard to complications, a 76-year-old woman with syncope at onset, fell and hit her head, had acute subdural hematoma the day after PMT

FIG. 3. *Upper*, Fountain infusion system; *lower*, lateral view of left pulmonary arteriogram. *Left*, pretreatment, thromboemboli filled in lower lobe artery, middle lobe artery, A6, A9, and A10 (*arrowheads*); *right*, 1 h after treatment, thomboemboli have been almost completely lysed

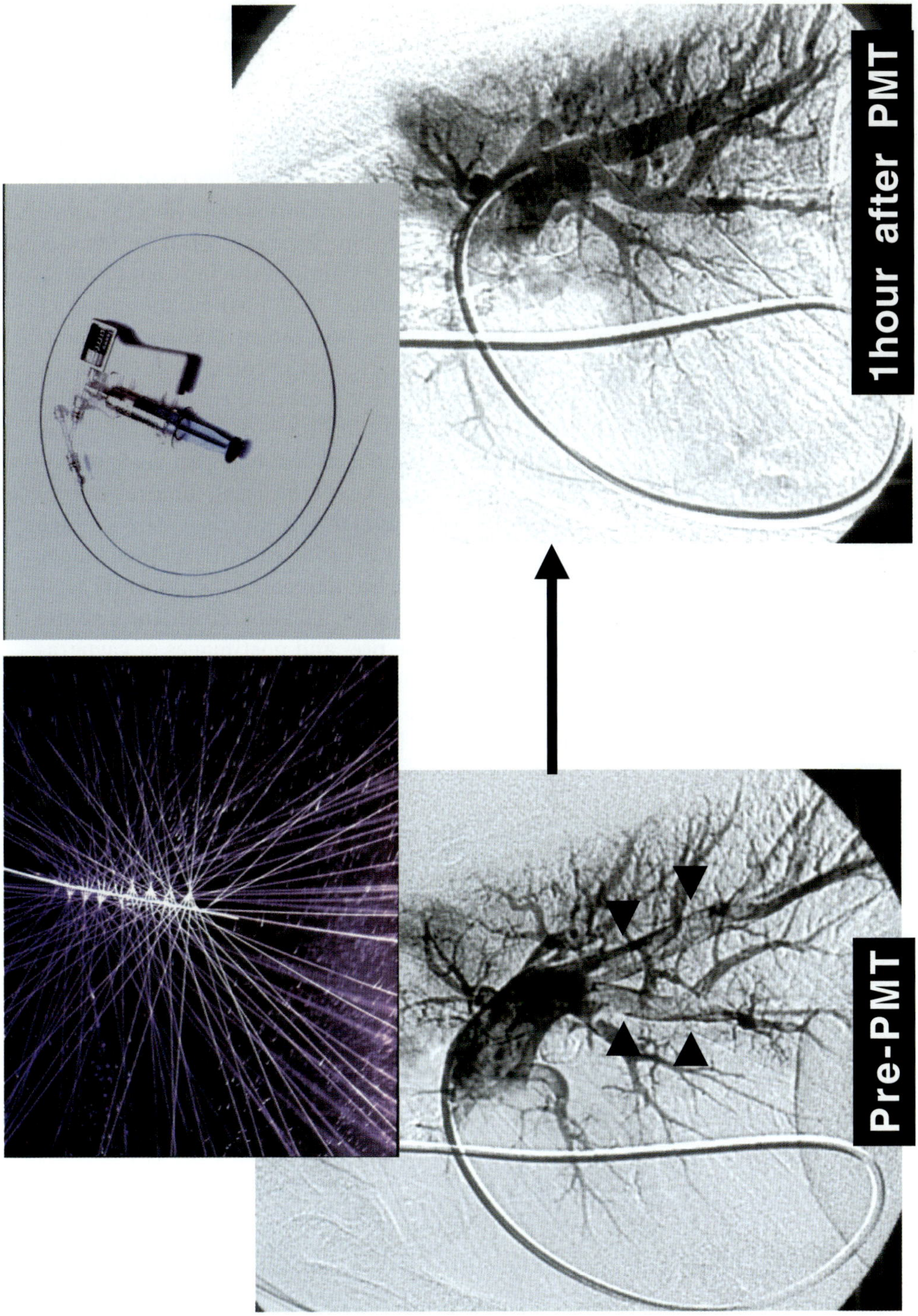
1hour after PMT
Pre-PMT

treatment began, and required surgical removal of the hematoma. There were no other serious complications or mortalities in either group.

Study 2

The time from DVT onset to the start of treatment was an average of 10.4 ± 7.1 days; the DVT was on the left side in 17 cases and on the right side in 6 cases. The most proximal veins with thrombi were inferior vena cava (3 cases), common iliac vein (10 cases), external iliac vein (2 cases), common femoral vein (4 cases), superficial femoral vein (3 cases), and subclavian vein (1 case). The PMT catheters were the Pulse spray catheter (E-Z-EM) for the initial 11 cases and the Fountain infusion system for the most recent 12 cases. The non-permanent inferior vena cava filters were the Neuhaus Protect filter (Neuhaus Laboratories) for 9 cases, the Antheor filter for 5 cases, the Filtrethery filter (Prothis) for 3 cases, and the Günther tulip filter for 5 cases. The filter was placed in the superior vena cava for the patient with subclavian vein thrombosis. The site of puncture was the popliteal vein (18 cases), femoral vein (3 cases), basilic vein (1 case), and internal jugular vein (1 case). The average total amount of urokinase used was 180 ± 127 units, and the average length of treatment was 4.5 ± 2.4 days. The VS score decreased significantly ($P < 0.0001$) from 20.0 ± 9.5 before treatment to 4.2 ± 4.0 after treatment, and the thrombolysis rate was 77.6% (Fig. 4). In the pre- and postimages of cavography, 3 cases showed capture of thrombi larger than 2 × 1 cm by the inferior vena cava filter, and removal was possible without symptomatic APTE after additional systemic thrombolytic therapy [6, 7].

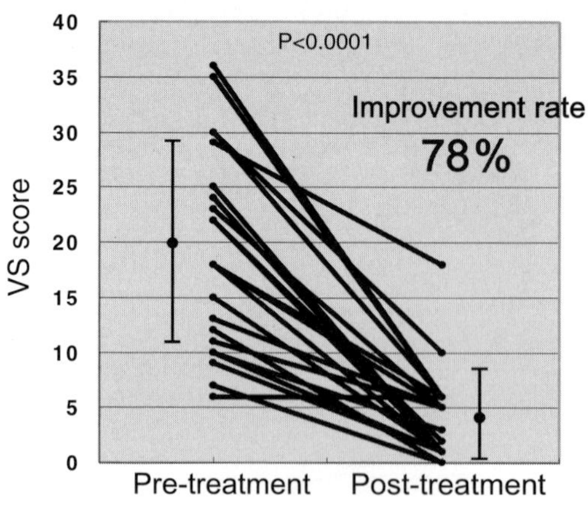

FIG. 4. Improvement of venographic severity (*VS*) score before and after pharmacomechanical thrombolysis for proximal deep vein thrombosis

Discussion

As a method of intravascular treatment of APTE, catheter-directed suction and fragmentation of the thrombus is used more frequently than catheter-directed thrombolysis at the present time, and studies suggesting its efficacy can be found in the literature [8–11]. Catheter-directed suction and fragmentation should be chosen with care in cases of total occlusion of the proximal pulmonary artery, in cases contraindicated for thrombolysis, and in cases where surgery is difficult. Efficacy and safety data, however, are still insufficient and there is the risk of deterioration of the hemodynamics due to distal thrombi when the catheter is repeatedly inserted in the pulmonary artery, particularly in severe cases. There are in fact reports of acute exacerbation during catheter manipulation [12].

With regard to thrombolytic therapy using catheters for APTE, a randomized study conducted by Verstraete in 1988 found no significant difference between rt-PA (recombinant tissue-plasminogen activator) peripheral administration and intraarterial administration in the improvement of pulmonary arterial pressure and pulmonary blood flow, from initiation up to 2 h of rt-PA treatment, and no difference in efficacy [5], and these results serve as evidence that there is no difference in the therapeutic effect between the modes of administration. However, with regard to PMT, which mechanically macerates the thrombus and makes lysis easier by spraying the thrombus forcefully with the medication, we found, not in a study of APTE but in a survey of efficacy and complications of peripheral venous administration and PMT, that an earlier thrombolytic effect was obtained in the PMT group. Furthermore, in the PMT method that we used for this study there were no cases of hemodynamic exacerbation, and we assume that by macerating the thrombus and inducing lysis at the same time the incidence of acute exacerbation should be lower compared to catheter-directed suction and fragmentation. In this PMT study, we have the impression that it was effective in regions with occluded large thrombi and poor blood flow. The number of subjects in the study was limited, so needless to say we should conduct a study with a larger number of cases in the future.

With regard to the treatment results of pharmacotherapy for DVT, anticoagulation therapy alone is reported to have yielded complete lysis in only 4% and partial lysis in only 14% of the cases, with the remaining 82% showing no improvement or deterioration [1]. Furthermore, with regard to thrombolysis of an occluded-type DVT, systemic administration from a peripheral vein produced only 14% complete lysis. In the case of catheter-directed thrombolysis, which has come to be used recently, it is reported that complete lysis was 72%, partial lysis was 20%, and swelling or pain of the lower extremities disappeared in 81% of the cases [2], showing that catheter-directed thrombolytic therapy is efficacious in achieving early thrombolysis [1–4]. According to a report by Mewissen et al. of a multicenter collaborative study on the effect of catheter-directed thrombolysis therapy for 287 cases, 303 limbs (71% iliofemoral vein, 25% femoropopliteal vein, and 66% acute-stage thrombus less than 10 days from onset), the results were 31% complete lysis (grade III), 52% partial lysis (50%–99%) (grade II), and 17% less than 50% lysis (grade I). The thrombolytic agent used was urokinase, the average total dose was 7,800,000 units, and the average duration of treatment was 53.4 h. The patency rate 1 year later was 79% grade III, 58% grade II, and 32% grade I, and the greater the thrombolysis the higher the patency rate [3]. Furthermore, it has been suggested that cases given catheter-directed thrombolytic therapy have a more favorable chronic-stage quality of life (QOL) compared to cases with anticoagulation alone [4]. Follow-up surveys have shown that cases with successful thrombolysis results have a low rate of postthrombotic syndrome and are able to maintain venous valve function [13, 14]. The difference in reactivity between new and old thrombi, in cases given catheter-directed thrombolysis, was 88% (160/181) in thrombi less than 4 weeks and 60% (15/25) in thrombi more than 4 weeks old. The prevalent method of catheter-directed thrombolysis in Western countries is the infusion method, which administers medication continuously from the catheter. With the PMT method used in the present study, highly concentrated medication is sprayed forcefully as well as applied directly, promising a mechanical effect on the thrombus. That mechanical effect may explain why, although the average dose of urokinase used in this study was much lower than the dose used in Western studies, we obtained similar therapeutic results.

Furthermore, in this study of PMT for DVT we found three cases with giant thrombi captured in their filters. Although there are reports in Western countries that inferior vena cava filters are not necessary [3], we believe that nonpermanent inferior vena cava filters are essential for APTE prevention when conducting thrombolytic therapy in the presence of acute-stage proximal DVT, particularly in DVT interventions [15–17].

Conclusions

No conclusions could be drawn from this study because of the limited number of subjects, but the results did suggest that PMT provides the possibility of earlier thrombolysis compared to peripheral venous administration in the treatment of APTE. In the future, we need to conduct a study with a larger number of cases.

PMT for proximal DVT is effective in achieving early thrombolysis, and the combined use of a nonpermanent filter made it possible to prevent the onset of APTE, a serious complication of intervention.

References

1. Comerota AJ, Aldridge SC, Cohen G, et al. A strategy of aggressive regional therapy for acute iliofemoral venous thrombosis with contemporary venous thrombectomy or catheter-directed thrombolysis. J Vasc Surg 1994;20:244–54.
2. Semba CP, Dake MD. Iliofemoral deep venous thrombosis: aggressive therapy with catheter-directed thrombolysis. Radiology 1994;191:487–94.
3. Mewissen MW, Seabrook GR, Meissner MH, et al. Catheter-directed thrombolysis for lower extremity deep venous thrombosis: report of a national multicenter registry. Radiology 1999;211:39–49.
4. Comerota AJ, Throm RC, Mathias SD, et al. Catheter-directed thrombolysis for iliofemoral deep venous thrombosis improves health-related quality of life. J Vasc Surg 2000;32:130–7.
5. Verstraete M, Miller GAH, Bounameaux H, et al. Intravenous and intrapulmonary recombinant tissue-type plasminogen activator in the treatment of acute massive pulmonary embolism. Circulation 1988;77:353–60.
6. Yamada N, Fujioka H, Ota M, et al. The efficacy of catheter-directed thrombolysis with temporary inferior vena cava filter for proximal deep vein thrombosis. Jpn J Phlebol 1999;10:307–15.
7. Yamada N, Nakano T. Catheter-directed thrombolysis. Jpn J Phlebol 2001;12:95–105.
8. Sors H, Meyer G, Reynaud P. Surgical and transvenous catheter embolectomy for acute pulmonary embolism: a review. In: Nakano T, Goldhaber SZ, editors. Pulmonary embolism. Tokyo: Springer-Verlag; 1999. p. 93–107.
9. Sharafuddin MJ, Hicks ME. Current status of percutaneous mechanical thrombectomy. Part I. General principles. J Vasc Interv Radiol 1997;8:911–21.
10. Greenfield LJ, Proctor MC, Williams DM, et al. Long-term experience with transverse catheter pulmonary embolectomy. J Vasc Surg 1993;18:450–7.
11. Schmitz-Rode T, Janssens U, Schild HH, et al. Fragmentation of massive pulmonary embolism using a pigtail rotation catheter. Chest 1998;114:1427–36.
12. Schmitz-Rode T, Janssens U, Hanrath P, et al. Fragmentation of massive pulmonary embolism by pigtail rotation catheter: possible complication. Eur Radiol 2001;11: 2047–9.
13. Arnesen H, Hoiseth A, Ly B. Streptokinase or heparin in the treatment of deep vein thrombosis. Acta Med Scand 1982;211:65–8.
14. Watz R, Savidge GF. Rapid thrombolysis and preservation of valvular venous function in high deep vein thrombosis. Acta Med Scand 1979;205:293–98.
15. Yamada N, Fujioka H, Yazu T, et al. Experience of temporary inferior vena cava filters. Sentan-iryou 1998;4:86–8.
16. Yamada N, Niwa A, Sakuma S, et al. Temporary inferior vena cava filters in Japan. Ther Res 2001;22:1439–41.
17. Ishikura K, Yamada N, Oota M, et al. Clinical experience with retrievable vena cava filters for prevention of pulmonary thromboembolism. J Cardiol 2002;40:267–73.

Thrombolysis During Cardiopulmonary Resuscitation in Patients with Acute Pulmonary Embolism

Fabian Spöhr and Bernd W. Böttiger

Introduction

Cardiac arrest carries a very poor prognosis, and few therapeutic options are available to improve outcome. In more than 70% of patients experiencing cardiac arrest, a massive pulmonary embolism (PE) or an acute myocardial infarction (AMI) represents the underlying cause of deterioration [1–3]. Acute PE has been identified as the immediate cause of cardiac arrest in 4.5% of patients with cardiac arrest studied within 8 years in an emergency department [4]. Therefore, acute PE is one of the most important causes of cardiac arrest. In patients dying of massive PE, the course of the disease is often both rapid and fatal; 40% to 90% of these patients have been reported to require cardiopulmonary resuscitation (CPR) within 1 to 2 h after the onset of initial symptoms [5, 6]. Conventional resuscitation procedures are rarely effective in fulminant PE unless pulmonary artery thromboembolism is treated immediately. Causal therapy options such as surgical embolectomy or catheter-assisted techniques are not readily available in all hospitals or in a prehospital setting. The use of thrombolytic drugs, in contrast, is established in most hospitals and has been shown to be an effective treatment option in patients without cardiac arrest suffering from acute PE [7]. In addition, thrombolysis has been demonstrated to be an effective approach for the treatment of cardiac arrest caused by acute PE [8]. However, it has not been regarded as a standard treatment for these patients. The major drawback to the use of thrombolytics during CPR has been the anticipated risk of severe bleeding associated with potentially traumatic resuscitation procedures such as chest compressions. Although not based on sufficient scientific evidence [9, 10],

Department of Anaesthesiology, University of Heidelberg, Im Neuenheimer Field 110, D-69120 Heidelberg, Germany

CPR has been regarded as a relative contraindication to thrombolysis by different medical societies [11, 12].

This review focuses on experimental and clinical evidence for and safety aspects of the use of thrombolytics during CPR in patients with acute PE.

Mechanisms of Action of Thrombolytic Therapy During CPR

There are at least two mechanisms that contribute to the effect of thrombolytics during CPR (Fig. 1). First, thrombolytic drugs act specifically at the site of coronary thrombosis or pulmonary emboli. Therefore, they treat the underlying pathological cause that contributes to more than 70% of cardiac arrests [1, 2]. Chest compressions during mechanical resuscitation may amplify the effect of thrombolysis, because thrombolytic drugs can act more effectively on blood clots that have been mechanically fragmented [13].

Second, experimental and clinical studies suggest another mechanism of action that may be of particular importance. After cardiac arrest, microcirculatory reperfusion failure is common and affects the outcome [14]. Although the pathophysiology of cerebral reperfusion disorders has not been completely understood, increased blood viscosity, endothelial cell swelling, leukocyte–endothelial interactions, and activation of coagulation with subsequent microcirculatory fibrin deposition and thrombosis have been reported to be important factors [15, 16]. This phenomenon, also referred to as the "no-

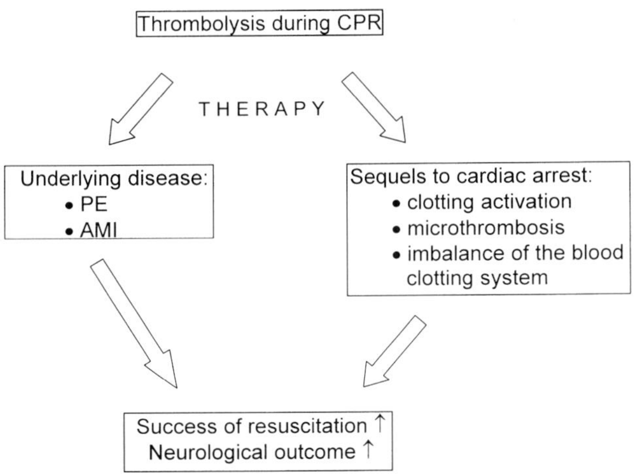

FIG. 1. Mechanisms of action of thrombolysis during cardiopulmonary resuscitation (*CPR*). *AMI*, acute myocardial infarction; *PE*, pulmonary embolism

reflow" phenomenon, prolongs cerebral ischemia and affects outcome after cardiac arrest. Experimental data demonstrated that cats receiving thrombolysis during resuscitation after 15 min of cardiac arrest showed a significant reduction of cerebral no reflow in the entire forebrain compared to untreated control animals [17]. These data are in accordance with results of intravital microscopy showing the occurrence of microthrombi in cerebral microvessels within minutes after the initiation of cardiac arrest [18]. Thus, experimental data have pointed out the pathophysiological importance of hemostatic changes for cerebral reperfusion and outcome of animals after induced cardiac arrest. As a consequence of these experimental data, it was hypothesized that an imbalance between coagulation and fibrinolysis may lead to microcirculatory fibrin formation and microthrombosis during reperfusion after cardiac arrest. In fact, an analysis of blood samples drawn during and up to 72 h after restoration of spontaneous circulation (ROSC) in patients with out-of-hospital cardiac arrest revealed a marked activation of blood coagulation in all patients. This was reflected in markedly increased levels of thrombin–antithrombin complex (TAT; a marker indicating the intravascular formation of thrombin) and levels of soluble fibrin monomers, a marker directly reflecting intravascular fibrin formation, during CPR. An elevation of TAT levels in patients with ROSC was found until 8 to 48 h after ROSC. In contrast, in most patients, the plasma levels of D-dimer, an indicator of endogenous fibrinolytic activity, were not markedly increased during CPR. It was concluded that in patients after cardiac arrest, a marked activation of blood coagulation occurred that was not counterbalanced by an appropriate activation of endogenous fibrinolysis [19]. These results were later confirmed by other authors who described massive fibrin generation with consecutive impairment of fibrinolysis during and after CPR in patients who suffered out-of-hospital cardiac arrest [20]. The activation of coagulation during reperfusion after cardiac arrest may be caused by hypoxia, stasis of the blood, endothelial cell damage, and high levels of catecholamines in the blood [16]. In addition, significant platelet activation was reported during and after CPR in humans [21, 22].

In summary, hemostatic disorders appear to be a major factor contributing to the impairment of reperfusion after cardiac arrest. Therefore, thrombolytic treatment may have two beneficial mechanisms of actions in patients with cardiac arrest (see Fig. 1). Both the direct actions of thrombolytics on coronary thrombosis or pulmonary emboli and the effect of thrombolytics on microcirculatory reperfusion may contribute to the exceptionally good neurological performance of patients even after prolonged resuscitation [13, 16, 18, 19].

Clinical Studies on Thrombolysis During CPR After Acute PE

The first report on thrombolysis during CPR in a patient with fulminant PE dates back almost 30 years ago [23]. Until recently, many case reports have followed, most of them demonstrating a dramatic success rate even after prolonged CPR and failure to restore a spontaneous circulation by regular treatment. Although case reports yield limited evidence, and the exceptional success suggested by these reports may, in part, be attributed to a selection bias in publication, outcome data were regarded as exceptionally good [9]. These case reports have been reviewed previously [13, 16].

In addition, a number of case series and clinical studies on thrombolysis during CPR in patients after massive PE have been performed (Table 1). Köhle et al. were the first to present a prospective study of 20 patients with massive PE requiring CPR. After pulmonary angiography, streptokinase was administered at the site of the pulmonary embolus. ROSC was achieved in 11 patients (55%) [24]. In a retrospective analysis, Scholz et al. reported a series of 9 patients with acute PE proven by angiography who received thrombolytic treatment during CPR. Seven of these 9 patients could be hemodynamically stabilized, and 5 patients survived. The duration of CPR was remarkably long; the times to reach ROSC were up to 90 min. The authors concluded that high-dose thrombolysis may be an adequate therapy option in patients with acute PE even during CPR [25]. Kürkciyan et al. retrospectively compared a group of 21 patients presenting with cardiac arrest after massive PE who were treated with a bolus dose of recombinant tissue plasminogen activator (alteplase) during CPR with a control group of 21 patients receiving standard treatment for cardiac arrest after massive PE. The number of patients with ROSC was significantly higher in the thrombolysis group compared to the nonthrombolyis group (17 versus 9, $P < 0.05$). The number of survivors, however, was not significantly different in both groups (2 versus 1) [4].

In conclusion, clinical studies and case series suggest a significantly improved rate of ROSC in patients with cardiac arrest due to massive PE and also a markedly improved long-term survival (54.3%) compared to patients receiving standard treatment in hospital (approximately 15% survivors [26, 27]). Moreover, most survivors had no severe neurological impairment after CPR, although resuscitation procedures were often longer than 90 min [13].

Out-of-Hospital Studies

Out-of-hospital studies on thrombolysis during CPR refer to a group of patients with a exceptionally poor prognosis. It has been estimated that only about 5% of patients with out-of-hospital cardiac arrest survive without

Table 1. Thrombolysis during cardiopulmonary resuscitation (CPR) in patients with acute pulmonary embolism (PE)

Reference	Study type	Number of patients	Thrombolytic agent	CPR-related bleeding	Number of survivors
Köhle 1984 [24]	Prospective	20	SK	—	11
Scholz 1990 [25]	Retrospective	9	SK/UK/rt-PA	Pectoral/sternal hemorrhage, liver laceration	5
Horstkotte 1990 [34]	Retrospective	17	UK	Two hemothoraces, liver hemorrhage	12
Siebenlist 1990 [41]	Case series	2	rt-PA	—	2
Böttiger 1991 [42]	Case series	2	UK	Liver contusion	2
Hopf 1991 [43]	Case series	7	rt-PA	—	6
Sigmund 1991 [44]	Case series	2	SK/rt-PA	—	2
Westhoff-Bleck 1991 [45]	Case series	5	rt-PA	—	3
Scheeren 1994 [46]	Case series	3	rt-PA	—	2
Kürkciyan 2000 [4]	Retrospective	21	rt-PA	Two liver ruptures, mediastinal bleeding	2
Ruiz-Bailèn 2001 [47]	Case series	6	rt-PA	—	4
Total		94		9 (9.6%)	51 (54.3%)

rt-PA, recombinant tissue plasminogen activator (alteplase); SK, streptokinase; UK, urokinase

severe neurological impairment [9]. Conventional CPR is not successful in most of these patients [28]. In most cases, the exact cause for cardiac arrest is unclear when the emergency medical service team arrives at the site where the patient had collapsed. However, because AMI and massive PE are the causes for more than 70% of patients who experience cardiac arrest, thrombolysis may be considered in the majority of patients with out-of-hospital cardiac arrest, unless the medical history strongly suggests another cause of cardiac arrest such as trauma or internal bleeding [29].

Up to now, four studies on out-of-hospital thrombolysis with a total of 299 patients have been published (Table 2). In the first of these studies, Klefisch and colleagues performed thrombolysis in 34 patients with suspected acute MI or massive PE during CPR in an out-of-hospital setting. This therapy was regarded a "rescue thrombolysis" in patients refractory to conventional advanced cardiac life support. Five of these patients survived longer than 3 weeks, 3 of them without neurological deficit [30]. In a prospective study that was performed at our department, 40 patients with out-of-hospital cardiac arrest received thrombolytic treatment with recombinant tissue plasminogen activator (rt-PA) and heparin during CPR after resuscitation had been unsuccessful for more than 15 min. Fifty other patients with comparable demographic data served as controls. Compared to the control group, significantly more patients could be hemodynamically stabilized in the thrombolysis group (68% versus 44%), and were admitted to an intensive care unit (58% versus 30%); 15% of the patients treated with rt-PA were discharged from the

TABLE 2. Thrombolysis during CPR: out-of-hospital studies

Reference	Study type	Number of patients	Thrombolytic agent	CPR-related bleeding	Number of survivors
Klefisch 1995 [30]		34	SK	Hemothorax	5
Böttiger 2001 [29]	Prospective, controlled	40	rt-PA	—	6
Lederer 2001 [31]	Prospective	108	rt-PA	Two pericardial tamponades, one hemothorax	27
Abu-Laban 2002 [32]	Prospective, randomized, controlled	117	rt-PA	One pulmonary hemorrhage, one major hemorrhage (not clearly specified)	1
Total		299		6 (2.0%)	39 (13.0%)

hospital alive, whereas in the control group, only 8% were discharged [29]. A retrospective chart review by Lederer and colleagues confirmed these data. Of 108 patients with out-of-hospital cardiac arrest who received rt-PA during CPR, 52 patients (48.1%) survived the first 24h and 27 patients (27%) survived to discharge. There was a significant improvement of outcome compared to a control group that was treated with conventional CPR (15.4% survivors) [31]. In contrast, the first randomized, double-blind, placebo-controlled trial on out-of-hospital thrombolysis during cardiac arrest did not show an improved survival of patients with pulseless electrical activity of the heart who were treated with rt-PA [32]. The studied patients with pulseless electrical activity, more than one-third of them having had no witnessed collapse, are known to have an extremely bad prognosis per se [33]. In fact, the outcome of the control group that was treated with conventional CPR was 0%, which means that there was not a single survivor among 116 control patients receiving conventional advanced cardiac life support. In this study population, even a therapeutic approach with proven efficiacy, such as hypothermia, would probably have failed [33].

In conclusion, data from the first studies on thrombolysis during CPR after out-of-hospital cardiac arrest are promising because they suggest a beneficial effect of this treatment on outcome and potentially even on neurological performance of survivors.

Differential Diagnosis of PE During CPR?

In an emergency situation, the exact cause of cardiac arrest can often hardly be established because of the short survival period of patients with acute PE. However, in some cases a typical medical history, a recent ECG, chest radiograph, or blood gas analysis that might have been performed at the beginning of symptoms of the patient could help to rule out other pathological conditions such as myocardial infarction, acute heart failure, cardiac tamponade, tension pneumothorax, or aortic aneurysm [8]. Echocardiography may be a useful tool for the diagnosis of PE even during resuscitation [34, 35]. Thrombolytic therapy will most probably have no beneficial effects in patients with cardiac arrest due to a ruptured aortic aneurysm or an intracranial bleeding. However, it should be considered that these patients—if they are in cardiac arrest—have an exceptionally poor prognosis a priori that is not likely to be affected by thrombolytic treatment [13]. In contrast, because AMI is the major differential diagnosis to massive PE in a patient with cardiac arrest [1, 2], thrombolytic therapy may improve the outcome of the patient even if a differential diagnosis between AMI and PE cannot be readily performed. Therefore, it might be indicated in many clinical situations to treat a patient with thrombolytic agents during CPR even without a final proof of the diagnosis. Such decisions should always be performed on an individual basis.

Bleeding Complications After Thrombolysis During CPR

The major safety concern associated with the use of thrombolytics is the risk of causing severe hemorrhagic complications. To estimate the risk caused by the combination of CPR and thrombolysis, it is important to classify bleeding complications, because both thrombolysis and CPR can cause significant bleeding complications even if they are not combined [10].

Bleeding complications are not unusual after conventional CPR [36]. Among CPR-related bleedings, hemorrhages of the heart and the great vessels, the lung, and abdominal bleedings are most common [28, 37]. Different autopsy studies [28, 36, 38] suggested hemorrhagic complications to occur in more than 15% of all patients after CPR [10].

It is well established that thrombolysis itself increases the risk of bleeding. In a meta-analysis of nine large randomized trials on thrombolysis for treatment of acute MI, the risk for major bleedings, defined as bleedings that required transfusion or were life threatening, was estimated to be 1.1% within the first 35 days after thrombolysis, compared to a risk of 0.4% in the control group. In addition, the incidence of intracranial bleeding after thrombolysis for acute MI was 0.8% compared to 0.1% in the control group without thrombolysis [39]. The incidence of intracranial bleeding after thrombolysis for massive PE may be up to 1.9%, one-third of them being fatal [40]. The risk for severe bleeding in patients with acute MI or PE who received thrombolytics can be estimated to be between 1.9% and 3.0% even without CPR as compared to 0.5% in patients not receiving thrombolytics [10]. Therefore, the important question is if CPR-related bleedings are more frequent or aggravated by thrombolysis.

Retrospective studies on thrombolysis shortly *after* CPR suggest that the incidence of severe CPR-related bleeding complications is comparable with the incidence of severe hemorrhage reported in the large studies on thrombolysis for acute MI or PE. An analysis of eight retrospective studies including 379 patients who received thrombolysis either shortly before or shortly after CPR revealed a risk of 1.1% for severe CPR-related bleeding complications [10].

The incidence of CPR-related bleeding complications reported by several in-hospital studies on thrombolysis *during* CPR in patients with massive PE appears to be higher than that reported in studies on thrombolysis *after* CPR (see Table 1). Eleven studies including 94 patients showed CPR-related bleeding complications in 9 cases (9.6%). Although these hemorrhages were considered to be severe, no patient died as a result of bleeding. Instead, the complications could be treated by blood transfusion or urgent surgical intervention [4, 25]. No fatal bleedings that were related to CPR have been reported in any of the in-hospital studies on thrombolysis during CPR in patients after massive PE.

Under out-of-hospital conditions, a markedly higher incidence of bleeding following the use of thrombolytics during CPR might be expected because history taking and physical examination of the patient is often limited. Interestingly, however, in the four out-of-hospital studies on thrombolysis during CPR, the overall incidence of severe bleeding incidents related to CPR was reported to be 2.0% (see Table 2). Klefisch et al. reported the successful resuscitation of 5 of 34 patients presenting with cardiac arrest refractory to conventional advanced cardiac life support who were administered thrombolytics during CPR as a therapy of last resort. One patient showed a hemothorax after prolonged resuscitation (75 min) [30]. In their retrospective study with 108 patients, Lederer et al. revealed by autopsy 6 severe bleeding incidents in a subgroup of 45 nonsurviving patients, 3 of which were considered to be directly related to CPR (see Table 2). However, in the corresponding control group of patients treated without thrombolysis, there were 7 cases of severe bleeding. Thus, the incidence of severe hemorrhagic events was not significantly different between the two groups [31]. The recent study of Abu-Laban et al. finally reported a pulmonary hemorrhage in the sole surviving patient treated with rt-PA, and one more major hemorrhage that was not clearly specified [32]. Again, none of these severe bleeding complications in patients with out-of-hospital cardiac arrest was fatal. In summary, the overall incidence of CPR-related bleeding complications reported in the studies on thrombolysis *during* CPR does not suggest that thrombolysis during out-of-hospital resuscitation is likely to contribute to an increased bleeding risk.

Conclusion

Thrombolysis during CPR in patients after massive PE may be an adequate therapeutic option to improve overall and neurological outcome of this group of patients with a very poor prognosis. Thrombolytic drugs appear to have beneficial effects by both direct action on pulmonary emboli and improvement of microcirculatory perfusion. Clinical studies provide increasing evidence that thrombolytic therapy during CPR can contribute to a stabilization in patients with cardiac arrest caused by acute MI or massive PE. In addition, an improvement in the microcirculatory perfusion caused by thrombolytic treatment of patients with cardiac arrest may be a major reason for an improved neurological outcome.

Thrombolysis during CPR may increase the incidence of bleeding events, but currently available data suggest that these potential risks probably do not outweigh the benefits provided by thrombolysis during cardiac arrest. Regarding the poor prognosis of cardiac arrest and the urgent need for causal treatment options, it is now necessary to assess the effects and potential risks of this promising treatment in a large, randomized clinical trial.

References

1. Silfvast T. Cause of death in unsuccessful prehospital resuscitation. J Intern Med 1991;229(4):331–5.
2. Spaulding CM, Joly LM, Rosenberg A, et al. Immediate coronary angiography in survivors of out-of-hospital cardiac arrest. N Engl J Med 1997;336(23):1629–33.
3. Zipes DP, Wellens HJ. Sudden cardiac death. Circulation 1998;98(21):2334–51.
4. Kürkciyan I, Meron G, Sterz F, et al. Pulmonary embolism as a cause of cardiac arrest: presentation and outcome. Arch Intern Med 2000;160(10):1529–35.
5. Böttiger BW, Bach A, Böhrer H, et al. Acute thromboembolism of the lung. Clinical picture–pathophysiology–diagnosis–therapy. Anaesthesist 1993;42(2):55–73.
6. Stein PD, Henry JW. Prevalence of acute pulmonary embolism among patients in a general hospital and at autopsy. Chest 1995;108(4):978–81.
7. Wood KE. Major pulmonary embolism: review of a pathophysiologic approach to the golden hour of hemodynamically significant pulmonary embolism. Chest 2002; 121(3):877–905.
8. Böttiger BW, Böhrer H, Bach A, et al. Bolus injection of thrombolytic agents during cardiopulmonary resuscitation for massive pulmonary embolism. Resuscitation 1994; 28(1):45–54.
9. Newman DH, Greenwald I, Callaway CW. Cardiac arrest and the role of thrombolytic agents. Ann Emerg Med 2000;35(5):472–80.
10. Spöhr F, Böttiger BW. Safety of thrombolysis during cardiopulmonary resuscitation. Drug Saf 2003;26(6):367–79.
11. Acute myocardial infarction: pre-hospital and in-hospital management. The Task Force on the Management of Acute Myocardial Infarction of the European Society of Cardiology. Eur Heart J 1996;17(1):43–63.
12. Ryan TJ, Antman EM, Brooks NH, et al. 1999 update: ACC/AHA guidelines for the management of patients with acute myocardial infarction: executive summary and recommendations. A report of the American College of Cardiology/American Heart Association Task Force on Practice Guidelines (Committee on Management of Acute Myocardial Infarction). Circulation 1999;100(9):1016–30.
13. Padosch SA, Motsch J, Böttiger BW. Thrombolysis during cardiopulmonary resuscitation. Anaesthesist 2002;51:516–32.
14. Hossmann KA. Ischemia-mediated neuronal injury. Resuscitation 1993;26(3):225–35.
15. Gando S, Nanzaki S, Morimoto Y, et al. Out-of-hospital cardiac arrest increases soluble vascular endothelial adhesion molecules and neutrophil elastase associated with endothelial injury. Intensive Care Med 2000;26(1):38–44.

16. Böttiger BW, Martin E. Thrombolytic therapy during cardiopulmonary resuscitation and the role of coagulation activation after cardiac arrest. Curr Opin Crit Care 2001; 7(3):176–83.
17. Fischer M, Böttiger BW, Popov-Cenic S, et al. Thrombolysis using plasminogen activator and heparin reduces cerebral no-reflow after resuscitation from cardiac arrest: an experimental study in the cat. Intensive Care Med 1996;22(11):1214–23.
18. Mossakowski MJ, Lossinsky AS, Pluta R, et al. Abnormalities of the blood–brain barrier in global cerebral ischemia in rats due to experimental cardiac arrest. Acta Neurochir Suppl (Wien) 1994;60:274–6.
19. Böttiger BW, Motsch J, Böhrer H, et al. Activation of blood coagulation after cardiac arrest is not balanced adequately by activation of endogenous fibrinolysis. Circulation 1995;92(9):2572–8.
20. Gando S, Kameue T, Nanzaki S, et al. Massive fibrin formation with consecutive impairment of fibrinolysis in patients with out-of-hospital cardiac arrest. Thromb Haemostasis 1997;77:278–82.
21. Böttiger BW, Böhrer H, Böker T, et al. Platelet Factor 4 release in patients undergoing cardiopulmonary resuscitation: can reperfusion be impaired by platelet aggregation? Acta Anaesthesiol Scand 1996;40:631–5.
22. Gando S, Kameue T, Nanzaki S, et al. Platelet activation with massive formation of thromboxane A2 during and after cardiopulmonary resuscitation. Intensive Care Med 1997;23(1):71–6.
23. Renkes-Hegendörfer U, Herrmann K. Successful treatment of a case of fulminant massive pulmonary embolism with streptokinase. Anaesthesist 1974;23:500–1.
24. Köhle W, Pindur G, Stauch M, et al. Hochdosierte Streptokinasetherapie bei fulminanter Lungenarterienembolie. Anaesthesist 1984;33:469.
25. Scholz KH, Hilmer T, Schuster S, et al. Thrombolysis in resuscitated patients with pulmonary embolism. Dtsch Med Wochenschr 1990;115(24):930–5.
26. Bedell SE, Delbanco TL, Cook EF, et al. Survival after cardiopulmonary resuscitation in the hospital. N Engl J Med 1983;309(10):569–76.
27. Ballew KA, Philbrick JT, Caven DE, et al. Predictors of survival following in-hospital cardiopulmonary resuscitation. A moving target. Arch Intern Med 1994;154(21): 2426–32.
28. Bedell SE, Fulton EJ. Unexpected findings and complications at autopsy after cardiopulmonary resuscitation (CPR). Arch Intern Med 1986;146(9):1725–8.
29. Böttiger BW, Bode C, Kern S, et al. Efficacy and safety of thrombolytic therapy after initially unsuccessful cardiopulmonary resuscitation: a prospective clinical trial. Lancet 2001;357(9268):1583–5.
30. Klefisch F, Gareis R, Störk T, et al. Präklinische ultima-ratio Thrombolyse bei therapierefraktärer kardiopulmonaler Reanimation. Intensivmedizin 1995;32:155–62.
31. Lederer W, Lichtenberger C, Pechlaner C, et al. Recombinant tissue plasminogen activator during cardiopulmonary resuscitation in 108 patients with out-of-hospital cardiac arrest. Resuscitation 2001;50(1):71–6.
32. Abu-Laban RB, Christenson JM, Innes GD, et al. Tissue plasminogen activator in cardiac arrest with pulseless electrical activity. N Engl J Med 2002;346(20):1522–8.
33. Böttiger BW, Padosch SA, Wenzel V, et al. Tissue plasminogen activator in cardiac arrest with pulseless electrical activity. N Engl J Med 2002;17347(16):1281–2.
34. Horstkotte D, Heintzen M, Strauer B. Combined mechanical and thrombolytic reopening of the lung-stream-track with massive lung-arterial-embolism. Intensivmedizin 1990;27:124–32.

35. Hopf H, Grote B, Becker H, et al. Erfolgreiche Lysetherapie einer perioperativ aufgetretenen, reanimationsbedürftigen Lungenembolie mit rekombiniertem Gewebeplasminogenaktivator (rt-PA). Anaesthesist 1990;39:50–2.
36. Krischer JP, Fine EG, Davis JH, et al. Complications of cardiac resuscitation. Chest 1987;92(2):287–91.
37. Nagel EL, Fine EG, Krischer JP, et al. Complications of CPR. Crit Care Med 1981;9(5):424.
38. Powner DJ, Holcombe PA, Mello LA. Cardiopulmonary resuscitation-related injuries. Crit Care Med 1984;12(1):54–5.
39. Indications for fibrinolytic therapy in suspected acute myocardial infarction: collaborative overview of early mortality and major morbidity results from all randomised trials of more than 1000 patients. Fibrinolytic Therapy Trialists' (FTT) Collaborative Group. Lancet 1994;343(8893):311–22.
40. Kanter DS, Mikkola KM, Patel SR, et al. Thrombolytic therapy for pulmonary embolism. Frequency of intracranial hemorrhage and associated risk factors. Chest 1997;111(5):1241–5.
41. Siebenlist D, Gattenlöhner W. Fibrinolysis with rt-PA for fulminant pulmonary thromboembolism. Intensivmedizin 1990;27:302–5.
42. Böttiger BW, Reim SM, Diezel G. Successful treatment of a fulminant pulmonary embolism using a high-dose bolus injection of urokinase during cardiopulmonary resuscitation. Anasthesiol Intensivmed Notfallmed Schmerzther 1991;26(1):29–36.
43. Hopf HB, Flossdorf T, Breulmann M. Rekombinanter Gewebeplasminogenaktivator (rt-PA) zur Notfallbehandlung der perioperativen lebensbedrohlichen Lungenembolie (Stadium IV). Anaesthesist 1991;40(6):309–14.
44. Sigmund M, Rubart M, Vom Dahl J, et al. Successful treatment of massive pulmonary embolism by combined mechanical and thrombolytic therapy. J Interv Cardiol 1991; 4(1):63–8.
45. Westhoff-Bleck M, Gulba D, Claus G, et al. Lysetherapie bei protrahierter kardiopulmonaler Reanimation: Nutzen und Komplikationen. Z Kardiol 1991;80(suppl 3):139.
46. Scheeren TW, Hopf HB, Peters J. Intraoperative thrombolysis with rt-PA in massive pulmonary embolism during venous thrombectomy. Anästhesiol Intensivmed Notfallmed Schmerzther 1994;29(7):440–5.
47. Ruiz-Bailen M, Aguayo-de-Hoyos E, Serrano-Corcoles MC, et al. Thrombolysis with recombinant tissue plasminogen activator during cardiopulmonary resuscitation in fulminant pulmonary embolism. A case series. Resuscitation 2001;51(1):97–101.

2. Catheter Interventions and Surgical Treatment of Acute Pulmonary Thromboembolism

Surgical Treatment for Acute Massive Pulmonary Thromboembolism in Japan

Motomi Ando, Mitsuru Yamashita, Masato Sato, and Ryo Hoshino

Introduction

Acute pulmonary thromboembolism occurs when thrombi formed in deep veins, mainly of the lower extremities or in the pelvis, cause an acute embolism in a pulmonary artery [1]. The disease states are varied, ranging from nearly asymptomatic cases to sudden cardiac arrest [2]. In severe cases hypoxemia or pulmonary hypertension will progress, ultimately leading to respiratory failure or right cardiac failure. The disease is initially treated medically [3], but if the thrombi are massive and diffuse, or if circulatory collapse occurs, it needs to be treated surgically [4–8]. This chapter describes mainly surgical cases.

Treatment Policy for Acute Pulmonary Thromboembolism

Diagnosis of Acute Pulmonary Thromboembolism

Although many cases progress without any symptoms, there could be serious consequences if the thrombi are massive and diffuse. Therefore, prompt clinical diagnosis is critical. It is especially important to suspect this disease if patients show postoperative signs of chest pain or respiratory distress. Echocardiography, computed tomography (CT) scan, pulmonary arteriography, and RI (lung perfusion scintigraphy) are used to obtain a speedy and accurate diagnosis. Echocardiography and CT scan are useful in determining whether surgery is indicated.

Department of Cardiovascular Surgery, Fujita Health University School of Medicine, 1-98 Dengakugakubo, Kutsukake-cho, Toyoake, Aichi 470-1192, Japan

Determination of Treatment Policy

Once the patient is diagnosed, treatment is initiated with anticoagulant therapy or thrombolytic therapy [3]. With regard to the medical treatment of acute pulmonary thromboembolism, thrombolytic therapy has been effective in a large number of cases, dissolving or reducing thromboemboli so that very few cases require surgery. However, medical treatment must be carried out with caution and with the possibility of surgery kept constantly in mind, as there may be patients whose dyspnea or right cardiac failure are exacerbated, or who experience cardiac arrest, during thrombolytic treatment. Treatment of postoperative pulmonary thromboembolism is determined by the nature of the operation and the patient's overall condition, but surgical treatment should be considered immediately postoperative in cases in which there is the possibility of bleeding from the operative wound and medical treatment is difficult.

Indication of Surgical Removal of Thrombi

When acute pulmonary thromboembolism is diffuse, the bilateral main pulmonary arteries are rapidly occluded and most patients could die within hours after onset. Furthermore, many mortalities due to acute pulmonary thromboembolism are caused by circulatory collapse in the stage immediately after the onset and by early recurrence. Therefore, in cases of circulatory failure or shock the main objective of treatment is to recanalize the occluded pulmonary arteries as quickly as possible. Generally, the indications for pulmonary thrombectomy in this situation are (1) cases whose hemodynamics are extremely unstable and who do not respond to medication, (2) cases with angiogram or CT scan findings of obstructions over a wide area of the pulmonary arteries, (3) cases showing rapid progression of heart failure or respiratory failure, (4) cases in which thrombolytic therapy is contraindicated, and (5) cases with thrombi suspended from the right atrium to the right ventricle [4, 5].

Many cases that fall into sudden shock before this disease is diagnosed cannot be operated on. Postoperative cases or long-term clinical patients who experience sudden dyspnea or who show signs of hypoxemia or right ventricular dilatation in their echocardiograms should be suspected of acute pulmonary thromboembolism, and percutaneous cardiopulmonary support (PCPS) should start immediately at the bedside. Furthermore, if there are no fatal cerebrovascular complications, and circulatory collapse due to the thromboembolism is identified, pulmonary artery thrombectomy should be carried out. Patients may include some who have thromboembolism (subacute pulmonary thromboembolism) of more than 2 weeks duration. Such cases are difficult to treat with conventional thrombectomy and should be diagnosed and their surgical indication determined with care.

Insertion of Venous Filter

Another form of surgical treatment for acute pulmonary thromboembolism, apart from thrombectomy, is the use of a venous filter inserted into the inferior vena cava to prevent recurrent or fatal thrombi. There are temporary and permanent filters for the inferior vena cava. Cases that may turn fatal (cases with massive and deep venous thrombi after surgery) are treated with temporary filters; cases in which anticoagulant therapy is contraindicated because of gastrointestinal hemorrhage or complications, or cases with repeated pulmonary thromboembolism despite anticoagulant therapy, are treated with permanent filters.

Surgical Treatment of Acute Pulmonary Thromboembolism

Surgical treatment of this condition involves removal of the thromboemboli by transvenous thrombectomy or open thrombectomy.

Transvenous Thrombectomy (Catheter Intervention)

This is a method whereby the thromboemboli are removed by suction using a catheter inserted transvenously into the pulmonary artery [9–11]. Catheters used in this method are the Greenfield catheter [9], guiding catheter for percutaneous transluminal coronary angioplasty (PTCA), and the HYDROLYSER embolectomy catheter. This method can be used for patients in whom thrombolytic therapy is contraindicated, and there are many reports, such as that of Greenfield et al. [9], of its efficacy. Still, because of the ever-present danger of circulatory collapse, transvenous embolectomy should be carried out under conditions where open embolectomy or PCPS is possible.

Open Thrombectomy

With extracorporeal circulation using an artificial heart-lung, namely under cardiopulmonary bypass, the pulmonary artery is opened and the thromboemboli are removed. If the patient has respiratory failure or poor hemodynamics preoperatively, extracorporeal circulation is quickly initiated using the femoral artery and vein. In cases of shock in the ward where hemodynamics cannot be maintained, the patient is transported to the operating room with PCPS. In cases of circulatory collapse with this disease, the speed of initiation of extracorporeal circulation is the key determinant of survival.

As for the surgical technique, extracorporeal circulation is initiated after median sternal incision, incisions are made bilaterally in the main pulmonary arteries, and open thrombectomy is carried out. Thrombi of acute pulmonary thromboembolism cases, in contrast to the organized thrombi of chronic cases, are soft and rod shaped, and the removed thrombi are relatively new and red. Although it is preferable to remove the thrombi as peripherally as possible, remaining thrombi can be treated postoperatively by thrombolytic methods if the major central thrombi have been removed. If they include those of more than 2 weeks duration (subacute pulmonary thromboembolism) that are firmly attached to the pulmonary arterial wall, care must be taken not to injure the arterial wall during the thrombectomy. The surgery can take place with the heart beating, but cardiac arrest is recommended for cases with multiple small thrombi in the segmental arteries or cases with thrombi firmly attached to the arterial wall.

Results of Surgical Thrombectomy

The results of open thrombectomy to treat acute pulmonary thromboembolism are as follows. Gray et al. [4] reported an operative mortality rate of 29.6% in 71 cases; Meyer et al. [5] 37.5%, 96 cases; Ohteki et al. [6] 25%, 8 cases; and Gulba et al. [8] reported 23%, but the results are worse in cases with preoperative cardiac arrest. Ando et al. conducted extracorporeal circulation during open thrombectomy on 16 patients and were able to rescue 12 cases, an operative mortality rate of 25%.

Open Thrombectomy Results: Ando et al.

Cases and Surgical Methods

Ando et al. conducted surgical treatment for 16 cases of acute pulmonary thromboembolism as of October 2003 (Table 1), 7 men and 9 women, aged 28 to 81 years (average, 56 years). Categorized by causative condition, there were 3 cases recuperating after cerebral infarct, myocardial infarction, and heart failure, respectively, 4 postoperative cases (after coronary bypass, surgery for thoracic aortic aneurysm, surgery for abdominal aortic aneurysm rupture, and lower limb orthopedic surgery), 1 case after arrhythmia catheterization, 1 case with a gigantic ovarian tumor, 2 pregnancies, and 5 with unknown causes. Deep vein thrombosis was recognized in 11 cases, 9 cases received preoperative medical treatment but they all had acute cardiorespiratory failure and required surgery, 12 cases fell into a state of shock, 9 cases required heart massage, and 2 cases were given PCPS in the ward.

TABLE 1. Surgical cases of thrombectomy under cardiopulmonary bypass for acute pulmonary thromboembolism

Case	Age (years)	Sex	Preoperative condition	Shock	Postoperative complication	Result
1.	72	M	Cerebral infarct[a]	(−)	MOF	Dead
2.	34	M	Dyspnea on admission	(+)[b]	Cerebral damage (mild)	Alive
3.	37	M	Acute myocardial infarct[a]	(+)[b]		Alive
4.	60	M	Dyspnea on admission	(−)	ARF, liver dysfunction	Alive
5.	81	F	Postoperative of CABG[a]	(+)[b]	Cerebral damage, LOS	Dead
6.	49	F	Catheter ablation[a]	(−)		Alive
7.	41	F	Ovarian tumor, dyspnea	(+)[b]		Alive
8.	58	F	Dyspnea on admission	(+)	Tracheal bleeding	Alive
9.	53	M	Dyspnea on admission	(+)		Alive
10.	79	F	Dyspnea on admission	(+)[b]	Cerebral damage	Alive
11.	76	M	Postoperative of AAA[a]	(+)[b]	MOF	Dead
12.	38	F	Pregnancy	(+)[b]		Alive
13.	28	F	Pregnancy	(+)		Alive
14.	53	M	Postoperative of orthopedics	(+)[b]	Mediastinitis	Dead
15.	67	F	Postoperative of TAA[a]	(+)[b]		Alive
16.	63	F	MR, CHF[a]	(−)		Alive

[a] In-hospital stay
[b] Cardiac massage (+)

CABG, coronary artery bypass grafting; AAA, abdommel aortic aneurysm; TAA, thoracic aortic aneurysm; MR, mitral regurgitation; CHF, congestive heart failure; MOF, multiorgan failure; ARF, acute renal failure; LOS, low cardiac output syndrome

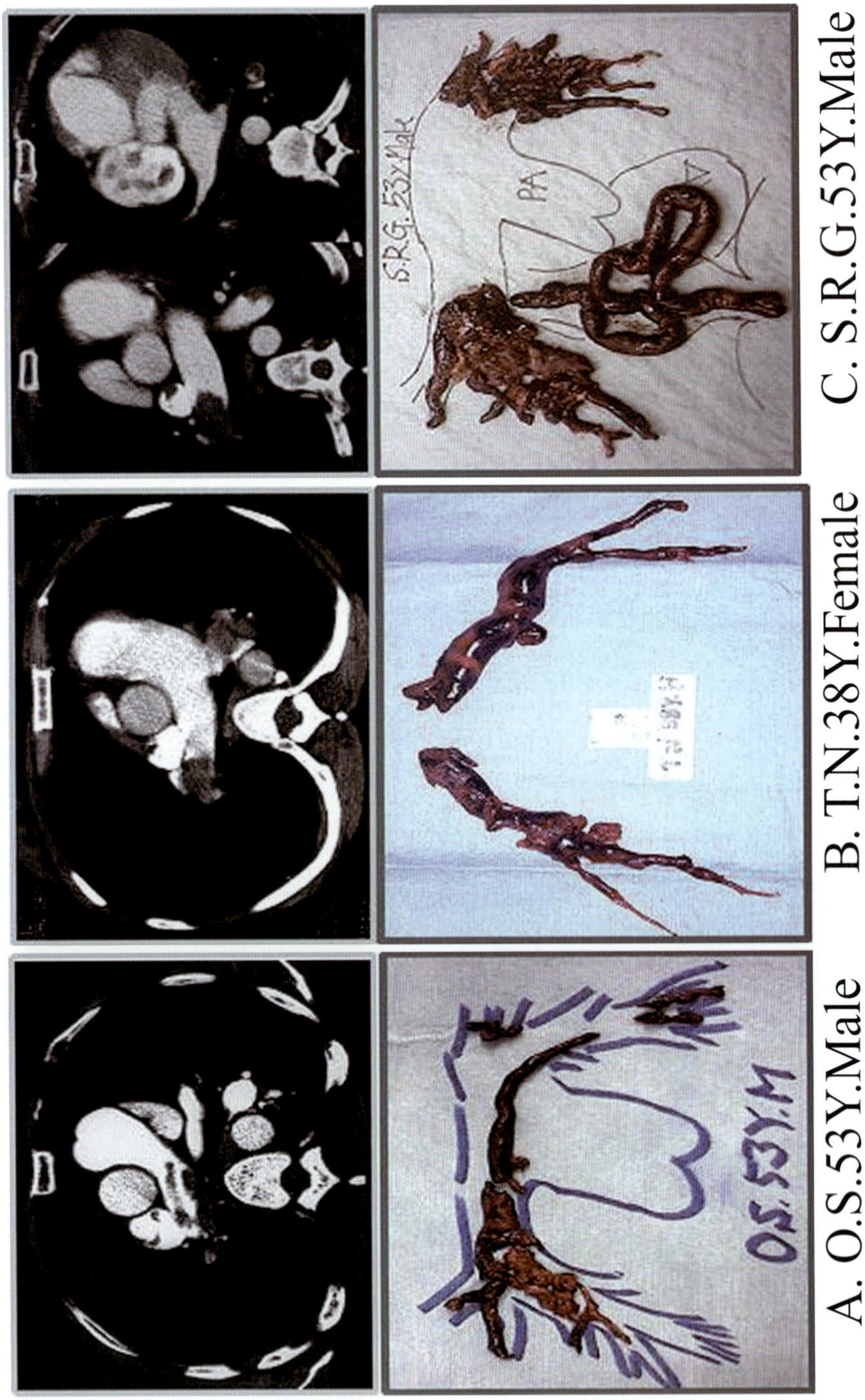

Fig. 1. Preoperative computed tomography (CT) and surgically removed thrombi. **A** A 53-year-old man, hospitalized with dyspnea and given emergency surgery. This case was a combination of acute stage and subacute stage of several weeks duration. **B** A 38-year-old woman, onset after cesarean section. **C** A 53-year-old man, onset after lower limb orthopedic surgery

As for the surgical technique, a median sternal incision was made, and under cardiopulmonary bypass, incisions were made bilaterally in the main pulmonary arteries and open thrombectomy was carried out. In the 12 cases of preoperative shock, extracorporeal circulation was quickly carried out using the femoral artery and vein before the median sternal incision; 6 cases had thrombectomy with the heart beating, and 10 under cardiac arrest.

Results of Surgical Treatment

Of the 16 cases, 12 showed a favorable postoperative course and survived. Case no. 2 had the postoperative complication of mild cerebral damage due to preoperative hypotension. The 2 cases that required PCPS died of a cerebral infarct and multiple organ failure, and cases 1 and 14 died in the hospital of multiorgan failure (MOF) and methicillin-resistant staphylococcus aureus (MRSA) mediastinitis (see Table 1). Inferior vena cava filters were inserted postoperatively in the surviving patients. Three cases of acute pulmonary thromboembolism are shown in Fig. 1. Prompt diagnosis by CT scan and thrombectomy under extracorporeal circulation were effective in all three cases.

Conclusions

We have reviewed the indications and methods of the surgical treatment for acute pulmonary thromboembolism, and presented our own results. When thrombi are massive and diffuse, or when the patient is in circulatory collapse, thrombectomy under extracorporeal circulation is extremely effective. Such cases require emergency surgery following a rapid diagnosis using echocardiography and CT scans.

References

1. Weinmann EE, Salzman EW. Deep-vein thrombosis. N Engl J Med 1994;331:1630–41.
2. Bell WR, Simon TL. Current status of pulmonary thromboembolic disease: pathology, diagnosis, prevention and treatment. Am Heart J 1982;103:239–62.
3. Konstantinides S, Geibel A, Olschewski M, et al. Association between thrombolytic treatment and the prognosis of hemodynamically stable patients with major pulmonary emnbolism: results of a multicenter registry. Circulation 1997;96:882–8.
4. Gray HH, Morgan JM, Paneth M, et al. Pulmonary embolectomy for acute massive pulmonary embolism. An analysis of 71 cases. Br Heart J 1988;60:196–200.
5. Meyer G, Tamisier D, Sors H, et al. Pulmonary embolectomy. A 20-year experience at one center. Ann Thorac Surg 1991;51:232–6.
6. Ohteki H, Sakai M, Akatsuka H, et al. Acute pulmonary embolism-diagnostic procedures, medical and surgical treatment (in Japanese). Jpn J Phlebol 1995;6:307–13.

7. Ando M, Tagusari O, Hanafusa Y, et al. Surgical thrombectomy under cardiopulmonary bypass for acute pulmonary thromboembolism (in Japanese). Ther Res 2000;21: 1131–3.
8. Gulba DC, Schmid C, Borst H, et al. Medical compared with surgical treatment for massive pulmonary embolism. Lancet 1994;343:576–7.
9. Greenfield LJ, Proctor MC, Williams DM, et al. Long-term experience with transvenous catheter pulmonary embolectomy. J Vasc Surg 1993;18:450–8.
10. Cho KJ, Dasika NL. Catheter technique for pulmonary embolectomy or thrombofragmentation. Semin Vasc Surg 2000;13:221–35.
11. Muller-Hulsbeck S, Brossmann J, Jahnke T, et al. Mechanical thrombectomy of major and massive pulmonary embolism with use of the Amplatz thrombectomy device. Invest Radiol 2001;36:317–22.

Emergency Surgical Pulmonary Embolectomy

Lishan Aklog

Introduction

Surgical pulmonary embolectomy has played a central role in the history of cardiac surgery. It was one of the first cardiac surgical procedures performed in humans, and it inspired the development the heart–lung machine. Despite its historical importance and the fact that its modern version was developed 40 years ago, its role in the management of patients with acute pulmonary embolism has been controversial. This controversy has persisted despite major advances in the safety and availability of cardiac surgery, our understanding of the biology of thromboembolic disease, and the emergence of alternative therapies such as thrombolysis and catheter-based embolectomy.

The challenge of determining the appropriate role for surgical embolectomy arises from the nature of the disease itself. Although acute pulmonary embolism is a fairly common disorder, it spans a broad spectrum of patients from those who are relatively stable to those who present in full cardiac arrest. Although the overall 90-day mortality rate has been reported to be about 15% [1], the actual risk in a given patient is directly related to the clinical presentation and the degree of underlying cardiopulmonary disease. In stable patients, without significant cardiopulmonary disease, this 90-day mortality can be well under 5% while patients who present in cardiac arrest have an in-hospital mortality of at least 50% to 60% even with surgical intervention [1, 2].

Given this heterogeneous picture, it is not surprising that pulmonary embolectomy has been so controversial. Skeptics tend to emphasize the overall operative mortality of about 30% reported in the literature while dis-

Department of Cardiothoracic Surgery, Mount Sinai Medical Center, 1190 Fifth Avenue, 1028, New York, NY, USA

missing the handful of reports with above-average results by saying that they included low-risk patients who should not have undergone surgery. Proponents, on the other hand, lament this nihilistic attitude and emphasize that embolectomy has become a relatively simple and widely available procedure which, if performed before cardiovascular collapse, provides immediate, dramatic relief of the obstruction with good short- and long-term results.

History

When Professor Friedrich Trendelenburg of Leipzig, Germany, presented his new operation for acute pulmonary embolism in 1908 [3], diseases of the heart and great vessels were still considered off limits to surgical treatment. He was motivated by the observation that, contrary to prevailing wisdom, most pulmonary emboli were not instantly fatal. He exposed the main pulmonary artery through a small left anterior thoracotomy, and the embolus was extracted with forceps through a small arteriotomy that was sutured closed under a clamp. Although he completed this procedure in less than 6 min, the patient died of hemorrhage from the back of the pulmonary artery. His two subsequent attempts were also unsuccessful. It was not until 1924 that his former trainee, Professor Martin Kirschner, performed the first *successful* Trendelenburg procedure.

Although Trendelenberg and Kirschner demonstrated that the hemodynamic insult of a massive pulmonary embolism could be reversed by direct surgical removal of the emboli, the operation did not enjoy widespread success. It was not until 1958 that the first successful Trendelenburg procedure was performed in the United States [4]. In their report they were only able to find 12 patients in the literature who had undergone successful pulmonary embolectomies.

In 1930, John Gibbon, a research fellow at Massachusetts General Hospital, was assigned to monitor the vital signs of a woman who developed a massive pulmonary embolism. She eventually deteriorated and an emergency Trendelenburg procedure was unsuccessful [5]. This vigil was the sentinel event that inspired Dr. Gibbon to spend the next 23 years developing a heart–lung machine that would have allowed ". . . some of the patient's cardiorespiratory functions to be temporarily supported . . . while the massive embolism was surgically removed."

Several modifications of the Trendelenburg procedure appeared in the 1950s, including pulmonary embolectomy during hypothermic [6] or intermittent normothermic [7] venous inflow occlusion. Although these techniques were a significant improvement over the classic Trendelenburg procedure, they were unable to salvage more than 30% to 40% of patients.

They are now primarily of historical interest except in the most desperate situations where a dying patient requires emergency embolectomy and cardiopulmonary bypass is not immediately available.

In 1961 Denton Cooley and Edward Sharp independently performed the first pulmonary embolectomies using cardiopulmonary bypass [8, 9]. The key elements of these procedures–cardiopulmonary bypass, pulmonary arteriotomy, complete evacuation of emboli under direct vision, and consideration of vena caval interruption—have been preserved over the past 40 years. These two successes led to a flurry of activity with multiple centers reporting on embolectomy with bypass in the next few years. The poor results from the classic Trendelenburg procedure and the lack of alternatives in this highly lethal condition made the 40% to 60% mortality rates in these early series appear quite acceptable. By the late 1960s and early 1970s, the basic techniques of embolectomy on cardiopulmonary bypass were well established. The debate on the indications for embolectomy, however, has continued to this day.

Major Surgical Series

Overview

We were able to identify 22 unique reports of at least 10 pulmonary embolectomies, incorporating a total of 837 patients, published since 1970 either in English or with a substantive English abstract (Table 1). Nearly all these series cover at least 10 years (mean, 15.7; range, 4–25) with the average center performing only 2.9 embolectomies per year (range, 0.8–7.1) and only four centers averaging more than 4 per year. The largest series averaged 7.1 procedures per year over 19 years for a total of 139 patients [10]. Three centers included a total of 100 patients undergoing embolectomy with the inflow occlusion technique [10–12]. The remaining procedures were performed on cardiopulmonary bypass.

Operative Mortality Rates

There were 261 operative deaths among 837 patients for an overall operative mortality of 31%, with nearly all centers reporting mortality rates of 20% to 40%. Although there is a trend toward slightly improved results in recent years, the operative mortality rate remains high (Fig. 1). It was 29% among reports published since 1990 compared to 35% for the older reports. It was 27% in those studies that only included patients since 1978 compared to 32% for those including patients from the remote past.

Embolectomy under cardiopulmonary bypass appears to have a lower operative mortality (29%) than with normothermic inflow occlusion (44%)

TABLE 1. Surgical series of pulmonary embolectomy

Lead author	Country	Publication date	Years covered	Number of years	Number of patients	Cases per year	Operative deaths	Operative mortality (%)
Aklog [51]	United States	2001	1999–2001	2	29	14.5	3	10
Doerge [13, 15]	Germany	1999	1979–1998	19	41	2.2	12	29
Ullman [14]	Germany	1999	1989–1997	8	40	5.0	14	35
Jakob [16]	Germany	1995	1988–1994	7	25	3.6	6	24
Gulba [46]	Germany	1994	1988–1993	5	13	2.6	3	23
Stulz [12]	Switzerland	1994	1968–1992	26	50	1.9	23	46
Laas, Schmid [17, 20]	Germany	1993	1975–1992	17	34	2.0	15	44
Meyns[18]	Belgium	1992	1973–1991	18	30	1.7	6	20
Bauer [19]	Switzerland	1991	1978–1990	12	44	3.7	9	20
Kieny [10]	France	1991	1970–1989	19	134	7.1	21	16
Meyer [21]	France	1991	1968–1988	20	96	4.8	36	38
Morshuis [22]	Netherlands	1990	1975–1988	13	16	1.2	6	38
Gray [23]	England	1988	1964–1986	22	71	3.2	21	30
Clarke [11]	England	1986	1960–1985	25	55	2.2	24	44
Jaumin [47]	Belgium	1986	1969–1984	15	23	1.5	7	30
Stalpaert [48]	Belgium	1986	1970–1984	14	29	2.1	10	34
Mattox [27]	United States	1982	1961–1981	20	35	1.8	17	49
Soyer [32]	France	1982	1977–1980	14	17	1.2	4	24
Glassford [24]	United States	1981	1969–1979	10	20	2.0	8	40
Tschirkov [25]	Germany	1978	1972–1976	4	24	6.0	7	29
De Weese [26]	United States	1976	1961–1975	14	11	0.8	7	64
Berger [49]	United States	1973			17		4	24
Heimbecker [50]	Canada	1973			12		1	8
Overall					837	2.9	261	31

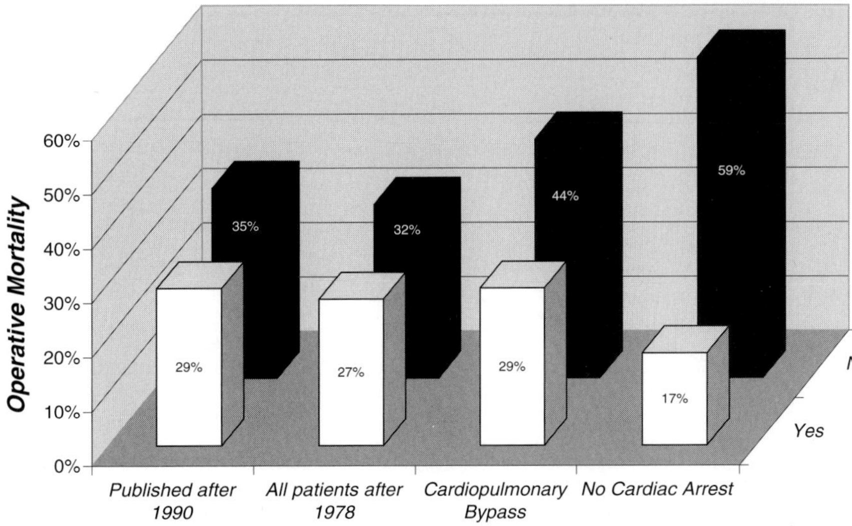

FIG. 1. Average operative mortality after pulmonary embolectomy in major surgical series listed in Table 1 as a function of publication date, inclusion of patients from before 1978, use of cardiopulmonary bypass (CPB), and preoperative cardiac arrest (CPR)

(see Fig. 1), probably reflecting the fact that, at most centers, inflow occlusion is used only in desperate situations. In fact, 46% of patients undergoing inflow occlusion had suffered a preoperative cardiac arrest, compared to 24% of the cardiopulmonary bypass group. Technical differences may also have contributed. Bypass provides more control, less time pressure, and better visualization than inflow occlusion and should permit a more complete embolectomy.

Risk Factors for Operative Death

Preoperative Cardiac Arrest

Among the 15 reports with preoperative hemodynamic data, the operative mortality among the 26% of patients who suffered a preoperative cardiac arrest was a staggering 59% [10–26]. The results in this high-risk group have not changed much over the years. It was 54% in the reports published since 1990 and 61% among those reports that only included patients since 1978. Although many of the remaining patients without preoperative arrest were in shock, their mortality was 17% overall and 10% if operated on cardiopulmonary bypass after 1978. Figure 2 demonstrates that operative mortality correlates fairly well with preoperative cardiac arrest. Hence, the centers that were

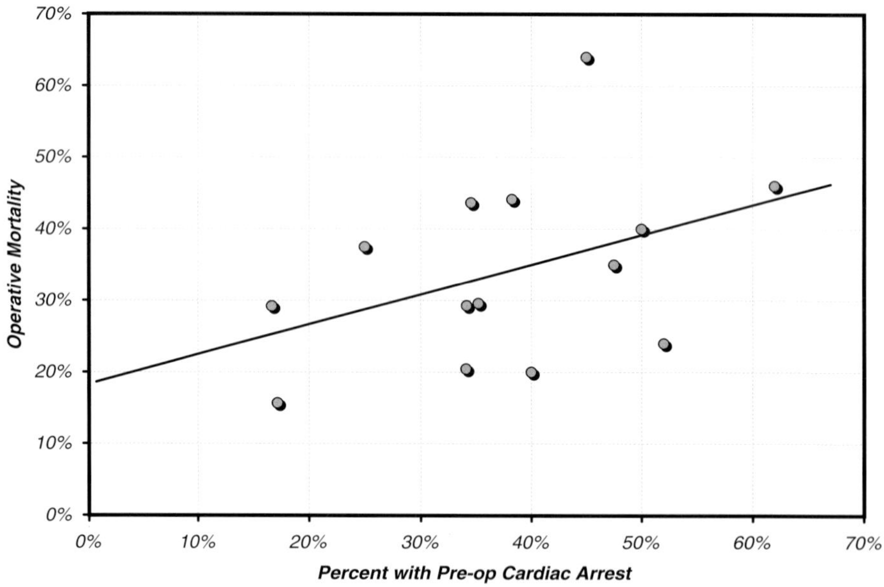

FIG. 2. Relationship between operative mortality after pulmonary embolectomy and proportion of patients presenting with preoperative cardiac arrest requiring cardiopulmonary resuscitation. Each *point* represents a published report from Table 1 that documents the preoperative hemodynamic status of the patient

able to operate before cardiac arrest generally had the best operative results [10]. Three of the more recent reports performed uni- or multivariate analyses to determine risk factors for operative mortality [12, 14, 21]. Preoperative cardiac arrest was clearly the most important independent risk factor, with odds ratios of 6.3 and 3.2 in the two multivariate analyses [14, 21].

Underlying Cardiopulmonary Disease

Both multivariate analyses also found underlying cardiopulmonary disease to be an independent risk factor for operative death, with odds ratios of 3.7 and 4.7, respectively [14, 21]. Patients with limited cardiopulmonary reserve are more likely to present with hemodynamic instability, shock, or cardiac arrest even with relatively low embolic burdens. They may be more likely to have smaller, more distal emboli, which are more difficult to completely extract. Increased pulmonary vascular resistance from incomplete embolectomy or underlying cardiopulmonary disease makes them more prone to postoperative right heart failure. Patients with normal heart and lungs, on the other hand, need larger, central emboli to develop significant hemodynamic compromise. These patients are therefore ideal candidates for embolectomy and can expect complete normalization of pulmonary artery pressures and right heart function.

Causes of Operative Mortality

Twelve reports document the cause of death after embolectomy [10, 12–14, 16–21, 23, 27]. Although these are not always well defined and the categories differ among studies, certain trends are clearly apparent. Figure 3a summarizes the leading causes of operative death in these studies.

Heart Failure

Heart failure accounts for approximately 44% of all operative deaths, with up to one-half of these resulting from failure to wean from cardiopulmonary

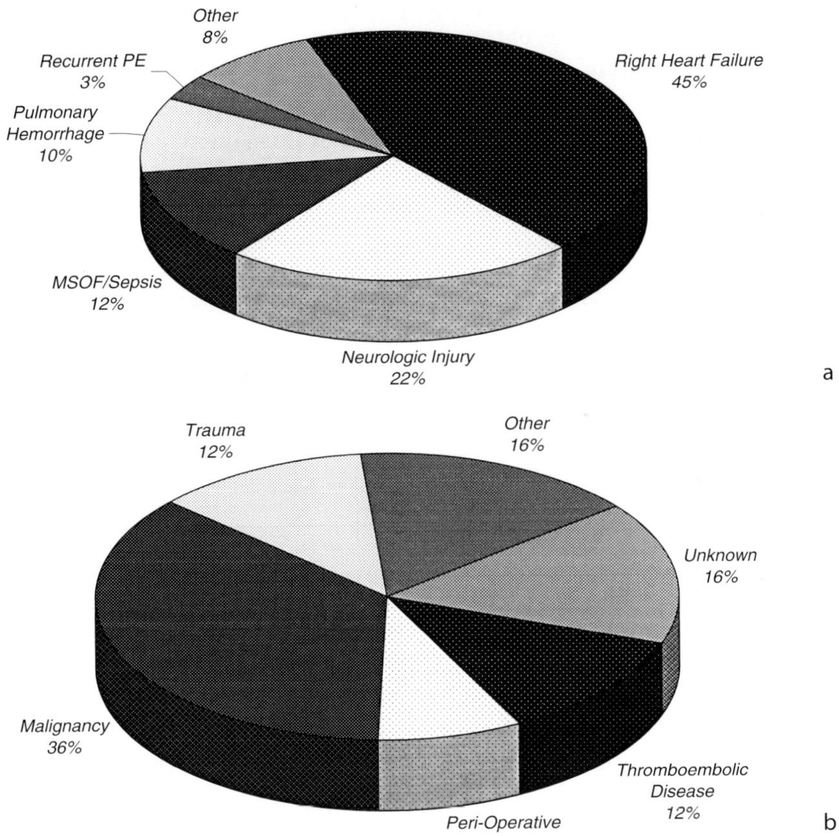

Fig. 3. Leading causes of operative (**a**) and late (**b**) death after pulmonary embolectomy in those major surgical series listed in Table 1 that report cause of death. *PE*, pulmonary embolism; *MSOF*, multisystem organ failure

bypass. Most of both the intra- and postoperative cardiac deaths are from *right* heart failure from severe preoperative right heart injury combined with underlying cardiopulmonary disease or incomplete embolectomy. Left heart failure only occurs in those patients with underlying heart disease, prolonged preoperative hypotension, or long aortic cross-clamp times. The risk of heart failure may be minimized by intervening before the onset of irreversible myocardial injury, assuring complete evacuation of all emboli, and avoiding aortic cross-clamping and myocardial ischemia, which may exacerbate the underlying myocardial injury. Operating on the beating, unloaded heart may be the best means of resuscitating the injured right ventricle.

Severe Neurological Injury

Severe neurological injury accounted for 22% of all deaths. This is usually a diffuse, anoxic injury resulting from preoperative shock or cardiac arrest with hypoxemia as an exacerbating factor. An occasional patient survives the injury but ends up in a persistent vegetative state. Intervening before cardiovascular collapse and aggressively treating with pressors to maintain adequate cerebral perfusion during the preoperative evaluation may minimize the incidence of neurological injury.

Multisystem Organ Failure and Sepsis

Multisystem organ failure and sepsis accounted for 12% of deaths. Many of these are probably secondary to prolonged pre- or postoperative low cardiac output. Maintaining adequate postoperative cardiac output with inotropic agents and volume during myocardial recovery is critical. Mediastinitis may also occur in an arrested patient undergoing sternotomy under nonsterile conditions.

Pulmonary Hemorrhage

Massive pulmonary hemorrhage accounts for 10% of deaths and is the only major cause of death directly attributable to the procedure itself. It typically presents as massive hemorrhage from the endotracheal tube with weaning from cardiopulmonary bypass [28–30]. Although some have attributed this to ischemia-reperfusion injury of the lung, the more likely cause is direct pulmonary artery trauma from overaggressive manipulation of the arteries or blind passes with forceps, suction tips or, especially, Fogarty balloon-tipped catheters; this can lead to pulmonary artery rupture and parenchymal hemorrhage or bronchial fistulization and massive hemoptysis. Blind clot extraction of any type is never necessary or worth the risk of this lethal complication.

Recurrent Pulmonary Embolism

Recurrent pulmonary embolism is occasionally reported as a cause of death, typically occurring within hours or days of the original procedure. It is poorly tolerated in these already tenuous patients, and repeat embolectomy is often futile because the second embolism may be a shower of small, distal emboli that are not easily extracted. The most common way to avoid this often-lethal complication is routine placement of an inferior vena caval filter.

Late Follow-Up

Patients surviving embolectomy appear to have a good long-term outlook, which is primarily determined by their underlying condition (malignancy, heart and lung disease, etc.) and not by their history of pulmonary embolism and embolectomy. Although formal follow-up is limited, a few studies do present data on causes of late death, actuarial survival, functional class, and follow-up diagnostic studies.

Survival Data

Ten centers report on 298 patients who pulmonary embolectomy and were followed for 16 to 127 months (mean, 71) [12–14, 16–21, 23, 31–33]. The 25 late deaths result in an overall late mortality rate of 8% and a linearized rate of 1.4% per year. Causes of death were documented in all 25 patients (Fig. 3b), and only 20% could be attributed to the history of pulmonary embolism: 2 following perioperative neurological injury, 2 from recurrent pulmonary embolism, and 1 from anticoagulation-related hemorrhage. Four deaths from unknown causes may have been related to pulmonary embolism. The majority of deaths, however, were from unrelated causes, mostly cancer (36%) and trauma (16%).

Recurrent Pulmonary Embolism

Clinically significant recurrent pulmonary embolism appears to be rare. Two patients, as noted above, died of recurrent embolism. There was only one additional report of a nonfatal embolism [19]. Although these retrospective studies might underestimate the incidence, they are consistent with the relatively low rate of recurrent thromboembolism in patients treated medically after pulmonary embolism [34]. In addition most, but not all, centers routinely performed inferior vena caval interruption to protect against recurrent embolism. The three patients who did suffer recurrent embolism had not undergone inferior vena caval interruption, either as a matter of policy [23] or for technical reasons [19].

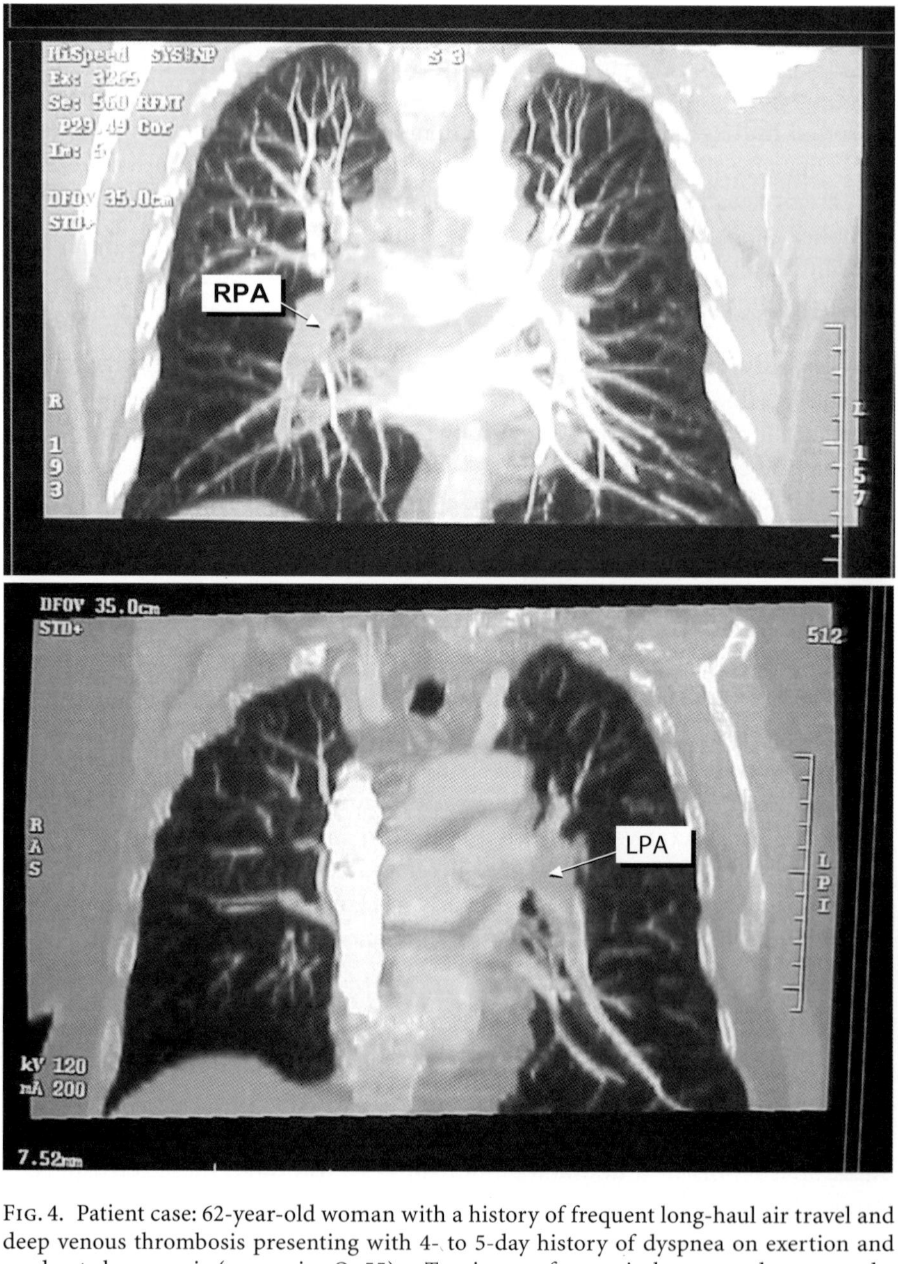

a

Fig. 4. Patient case: 62-year-old woman with a history of frequent long-haul air travel and deep venous thrombosis presenting with 4- to 5-day history of dyspnea on exertion and moderate hypoxemia (room air pO_2 55). **a** Two images from spiral computed tomography (CT) scan with coronal reconstruction obtained at an outside emergency room demonstrating massive saddle pulmonary embolism extending into both right (*RPA*) and left (*LPA*) pulmonary arteries. The patient was transported to operating room by helicopter without further testing. **b** Intraoperative photograph (*upper image*) taken from the patient's left side (the patient's head is toward the right) demonstrating the saddle embolus straddling the bifurcation of the main pulmonary artery (*MPA*). The right ventricular outflow tract (*RVOT*), ascending aorta (*Asc Ao*), aortic cannula (*Ao Cann*), and venous cannula (*Ven Cann*) are labeled.

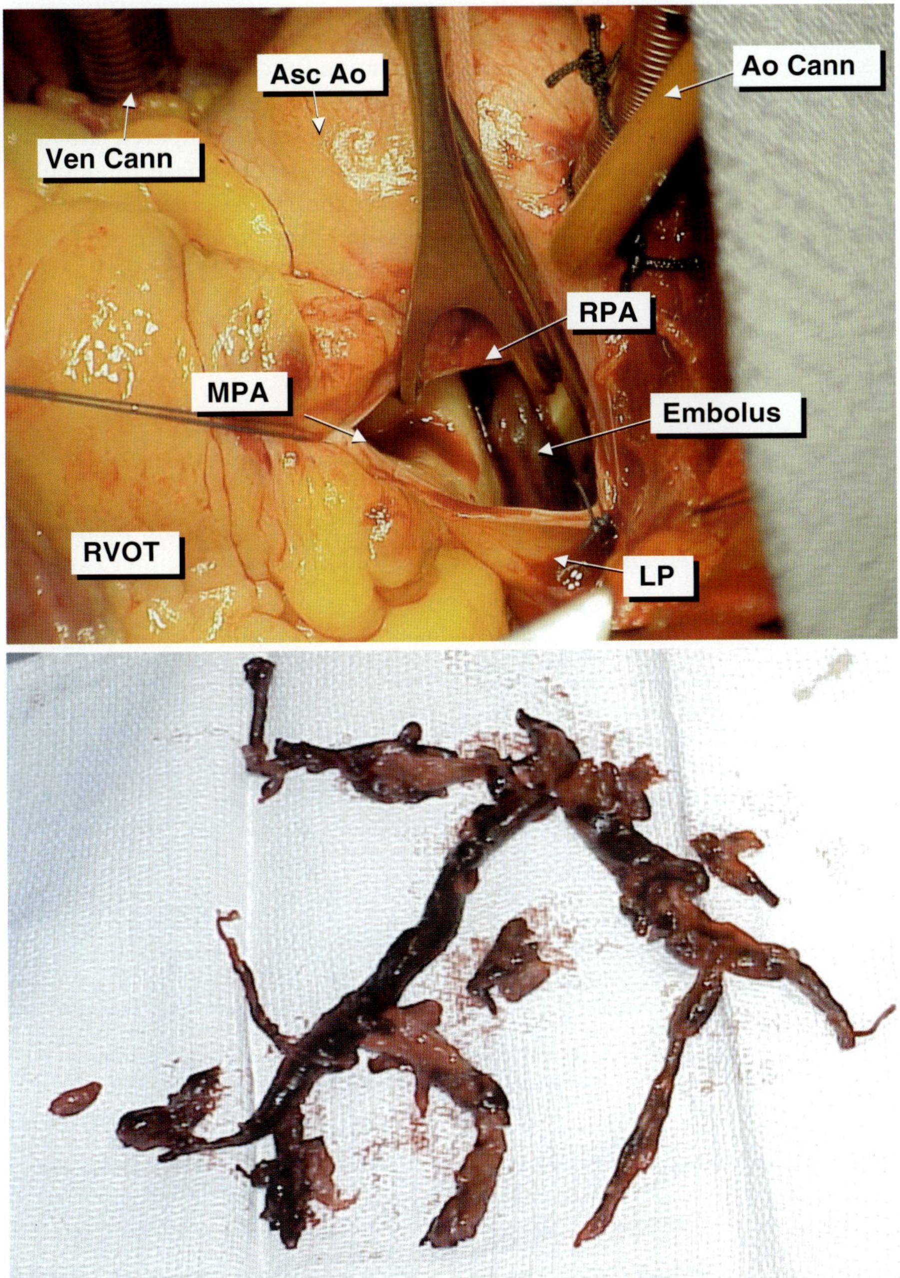

b

FIG. 4. *Continued*. The *lower image* shows the extracted thromboemboli in their approximate anatomic configuration within the pulmonary arterial tree. Several segments are clearly casts of the femoral veins, and their heterogeneous consistency suggests multiple embolizations over some period of time. Patient weaned off cardiopulmonary bypass easily, had an uneventful postoperative course, was discharged to home, and is doing well 10 months postoperatively

Functional Status

Six studies document New York Heart Association functional class in 176 hospital survivors at a mean follow-up of 71 months [13, 14, 19, 21, 31, 33]. Nearly all (98%) were in class I or II. One nonrandomized study compared late functional status among patients treated with heparin, streptokinase, or embolectomy [33]. Although the surgical patients were more ill at presentation, their late functional status was better, with 45% in class I compared to 17% of medical patients. No surgical patient was in class III or IV compared to 10% of medical patients.

Preoperative Evaluation

Surgical Indications and Timing

Overall Strategy

There is no consensus on the indications for surgery in acute pulmonary embolism (Table 2). The decision is fairly straightforward at either extreme.

TABLE 2. Factors to consider in the decision to proceed with surgical pulmonary embolectomy

Possible indications for embolectomy	Contraindications to thrombolysis	
	Absolute	Relative
Embolus in the central pulmonary arteries	Active internal bleeding	Age over 75 years
More than 50% obstruction of pulmonary vasculature	Intracranial neoplasm, vascular malformation, or aneurysm	Recent (less than 10 days) major surgery, puncture of noncompressible puncture, or organ biopsy
Refractory cardiogenic shock	Neurosurgical procedure or stroke within 2 months	Pregnancy or early postpartum
Right atrial or ventricular thrombus	Severe uncontrolled hypertension	Recent trauma, including chest compressions
Severe right heart dysfunction	Known bleeding diathesis	Recent gastrointestinal bleeding or active ulcer disease (less than 10 days)
Elevated cardiac troponin	Known allergy to thrombolytic agents	Known coagulation defects, including anticoagulant therapy and significant liver dysfunction
Moderate hemodynamic compromise or right heart dysfunction with contraindication to thrombolysis		High likelihood of left heart thrombus (e.g., mitral stenosis with atrial fibrillation)

A stable patient with multiple peripheral perfusion defects is clearly not a surgical candidate. On the other hand, a patient in refractory cardiogenic shock with a documented saddle embolus, and a contraindication to thrombolysis, is certainly best served by emergency embolectomy. Most patients, however, fall between these two extremes and require careful, individualized assessment to determine the optimal management. The indications for surgery should be part of a multidisciplinary strategy that seeks to minimize *overall* morbidity and mortality using all available modalities. Embolectomy should be considered one tool that, if applied before severe hemodynamic compromise, can provide excellent short *and* long-term results. A strategy that positions it as a treatment of last resort, to be avoided unless other options have failed or are unavailable, is doomed, in my opinion, to provide suboptimal results.

Location of Pulmonary Emboli

The classic anatomic criteria for embolectomy has been more than 50% obstruction of the pulmonary vascular tree by pulmonary angiography. The location of the emboli, however, may be as important as the degree of obstruction. The ideal surgical patient has large emboli in the central pulmonary arteries that can be completely removed in a few pieces, resulting in normalization of the pulmonary artery pressures and restoration of right heart function. A patient who has showered multiple emboli may also demonstrate vascular obstruction approaching 50% but is not a good surgical candidate. Complete embolectomy may not be possible in these patients without traumatic maneuvers such as massaging the lungs, blind passage of instruments into the periphery, or retrograde perfusion of the lungs through the pulmonary veins.

Hemodynamic Status

As we have seen from the results of the major surgical series, a specific center's results will primarily depend on its hemodynamic threshold for intervening surgically. If surgery is limited to those patients in extremis, one can expect mortality rates greater than 50%. If surgery is applied more liberally with every effort to intervene *before* the onset of shock or cardiac arrest, one can expect mortality rates as low as 10%, comparable to patients undergoing thrombolysis [35]. This dichotomy is understandable given that the leading causes of operative death—right heart failure, neurological injury, and multisystem organ failure—are a result of the patient's preoperative hemodynamic condition and not the procedure itself. Pulmonary embolectomy, if applied with attention to minimizing pulmonary artery trauma, is a relatively simple procedure that should carry little inherent risk of death. Cardiopulmonary bypass times should be short, cardioplegic arrest should be unnecessary, and bleeding complications should be minimal.

The fact that some patients will always present with sudden cardiovascular collapse may make it impossible to lower the overall mortality rate to less than 5% to 10% unless patients in extremis are simply not offered surgery. However, as Trendelenburg observed nearly a century ago, most patients have between 15 min and several hours before severe hemodynamic compromise ensues. Utilizing this time period effectively is the most critical challenge, with high stakes on both sides. Delaying surgery for a trial of medical therapy may avoid a major operation but may risk converting a stable patient with an operative mortality of 5% to 10% to one in severe cardiogenic shock or cardiac arrest with a mortality of 40% to 60%.

Sasahara's classic hemodynamic criteria for embolectomy include refractory cardiogenic shock and oliguria despite *maximal* medical therapy or when thrombolytic therapy is contraindicated [36]. These stringent criteria, however, may withhold a potentially life-saving procedure until irreversible cardiac and end-organ injury has occurred. In my opinion, all patients with a hemodynamically significant central embolus should be *considered* for surgery. If the patient stabilizes then thrombolytic therapy may be appropriate, but the surgical team must be kept on alert and notified early if the patient deteriorates. The use of high-dose pressors during thrombolytic therapy to avoid surgery at all costs is inappropriate.

Right Heart Function

Goldhaber and others have clearly demonstrated that right ventricular hypokinesis without systemic hypotension is a strong, independent risk factor for early mortality and that this finding can be used to triage patients to more aggressive treatment [1, 37]. This risk stratification has typically been applied in selecting patients for thrombolysis but may also be used in recommending embolectomy in those patients with contraindications to thrombolysis, even if they are hemodynamically stable. Evidence of *severe* right ventricular dysfunction might justify proceeding with embolectomy even if thrombolytic therapy is not contraindicated.

Right Atrial or Ventricular Thrombus

Mobile thrombus or "in-transit" emboli within the right atrium or right ventricle may occur in up to 10% to 15% of patients with pulmonary embolism [38, 39]. Even modest-sized thrombi can be fatal if they embolize in a patient with moderate degrees of vascular obstruction and right heart dysfunction. Because they are associated with a high (>40%) mortality rate, their presence is generally considered a strong indication for aggressive intervention. Although thrombolysis has been advocated for this condition [38, 40, 41], embolectomy may be the most appropriate treatment. These thrombi can embolize at any time [42], and thrombolysis can take several hours to achieve its maximal effect and might actually promote embolization. In my opinion, the presence of mobile thrombi in the right heart in a patient with documented central pulmonary emboli is a strong indication for emergency surgery.

Contradictions to Thrombolytic Therapy

Thrombolytic therapy has been shown to accelerate the resolution of emboli, the normalization of pulmonary artery pressures and right heart function, and lower mortality in selected patients [43–45]. The risk of intracranial hemorrhage is about 1% and the risk of other major hemorrhage is 10% to 20%. Some patients, however, have significantly higher risks of complications and thrombolytic therapy is contraindicated in them (see Table 2). Patients with central pulmonary emboli who would be candidates for thrombolytic therapy but have contraindications should be considered for surgical embolectomy.

Diagnostic Studies

Overall Strategy

A streamlined diagnostic approach, focusing on documenting central emboli as rapidly as possible, is critical to achieving good results in patients being considered for embolectomy. Once this has been done, the patient should be *immediately* transported to the operating room even if relatively stable. Echocardiography, pulmonary angiography, and computed tomography (CT) scanning all play important roles, but the specific tests performed depends on the patient's clinical presentation, location, and what is available to the clinicians. Although many patients will have undergone ventilation-perfusion scintigraphy at some point, this study is not particularly helpful in this setting. Large perfusion defects may suggest central emboli, but their actual location cannot reliably be determined without a chest CT scan or pulmonary angiogram.

Chest CT Scanning

Contrast-enhanced spiral CT scanning of the chest has become increasingly popular in the evaluating pulmonary embolism. It may, in fact, be the ideal study in emergency room patients with suspected major pulmonary embolism. Although spiral CT is usually necessary to document peripheral emboli, large central emboli are usually well visualized with a standard scan. CT scanning is usually readily available, often in the emergency room itself, and can be performed in 10 to 15 min. If central emboli are visualized in the main or proximal branch pulmonary arteries and the patient is a candidate for surgical embolectomy by clinical criteria, no further confirmatory testing is necessary and the patient can be immediately transported to the operating room.

Echocardiography

Echocardiography, transthoracic and transesophageal, is also playing an increasing role in the diagnosis and risk stratification of patients with pulmonary embolism. Although the pulmonary arteries themselves are often not well visualized, echocardiography provides important information that can confirm the diagnosis and determine whether aggressive treatment should be considered. Right heart function can be assessed, pulmonary artery pressures can be estimated, and mobile thromboemboli in the right atrium or ventricle can be visualized. As previously mentioned, right ventricular hypokinesis is a strong predictor of poor outcome and may justify aggressive treatment—thrombolysis or surgery—even if the patient is hemodynamically stable.

Echocardiography may also be helpful as an initial study in a patient with some hemodynamic compromise in whom the diagnosis of pulmonary embolism is being considered. If the echocardiogram is suggestive but not definitive, a confirmatory CT scan or, more likely, pulmonary angiogram would be indicated. A tenuous patient, with clear-cut echocardiographic findings of a major pulmonary embolism, who is considered a candidate for surgical embolectomy, could be taken to the operating room without further testing. Intraoperative transesophageal or surface echocardiography could then confirm the presence of central emboli.

Pulmonary Angiography

Although pulmonary angiography remains the gold standard for diagnosing pulmonary embolism, its role in evaluating patients for embolectomy should be limited. With spiral CT and echocardiography, most embolectomy patients will not need preoperative angiography. Clinically stable patients, with intermediate to high probability ventilation-perfusion scans, may undergo confirmatory angiography where unsuspected, massive, central pulmonary embolism requiring surgery is discovered. Other patients, with echocardiographic findings suggestive of a large embolism, might need angiography to define the anatomic distribution of emboli and to determine whether surgical embolectomy is appropriate.

Intraoperative and Postoperative Management

Basic Principles

Patients selected for embolectomy should be immediately transported to the operating room even if they "appear" relatively stable. In our hospital, patients go directly from the radiology suite or ward to the operating room without stopping in the intensive care unit for "stabilization." Resuscitation can be performed en route and in the operating room. Patients from outside hospitals are transferred directly to the operating room by helicopter. In the operating room, teamwork is critical and only essential preoperative maneuvers are performed so the patient can be placed on cardiopulmonary bypass without delay.

Anesthesia

Patients with large central pulmonary emboli are very tenuous, even if awake and relatively stable. The failing right ventricle is dependent on elevated preload to maintain flow through the obstructed pulmonary vasculature. The underfilled left ventricle is dependent on increased peripheral vascular tone to maintain systemic blood pressure. Although compensatory mechanisms can maintain normal blood pressure, small hemodynamic perturbations, such as venous and arterial vasodilatation from general anesthesia, can reverse these mechanisms and lead to hemodynamic collapse. Anesthesia should not begin until the perfusionist is present with the heart-lung machine primed and ready. Prepping and draping the patient before induction may also be prudent as this will allow the surgeon to open the chest and be on bypass within a few minutes.

Transesophageal Echocardiography

Intraoperative transesophageal echocardiography (TEE) is a useful tool during embolectomy. Imaging of the right atrium and ventricle before cannulation for bypass is helpful. Visualization of mobile thromboemboli in the right heart can help determine whether right heart exploration is necessary and guide venous cannulation. Assessment of right heart function can help anticipate difficulties with weaning from bypass. TEE can often visualize emboli in the central pulmonary arteries in a patient who has come to the operating room without good visualization of these structures. Surface scanning of the right heart and pulmonary arteries is very simple and can be used in the occasional patient who cannot undergo TEE or in whom adequate images cannot be obtained.

Surgical Technique

Incision and Cardiopulmonary Bypass

After full median sternotomy, pericardiotomy and full heparinization, the patient is cannulated for cardiopulmonary bypass. With vacuum-assisted venous drainage, the right atrium can be explored without separately controlling the vena cavae. Although some authors report using aortic cross-clamping and cardioplegic or fibrillatory arrest, this is, in my opinion, never necessary and potentially detrimental. Pulmonary embolectomy and right heart exploration can easily be performed with the heart beating under normothermic conditions. Performing the operation on the unloaded, well-perfused beating heart not only avoids any further ischemic insult to the stunned right ventricle, it also provides a period of time for the heart to recover and regenerate its depleted energy stores. If echocardiography demonstrates mobile thromboemboli in the right atrium or right ventricle, exploration of these chambers is mandatory and should be performed before embolectomy.

Pulmonary Arteriotomy and Embolectomy

Once cardiopulmonary bypass has been established, the actual embolectomy begins with an incision over the main pulmonary artery. The clot is then gently extracted, en bloc if possible, under direct vision using simple gall-bladder stone forceps.

Many other techniques for clot extraction have been utilized and advocated in the literature. I believe that these techniques are not only unnecessary but also excessively traumatic and potentially dangerous. The pulmonary arteries are very fragile, and trauma to these vessels from overaggressive or blind instrumentation can lead to pulmonary hemorrhage, which is usually fatal. If patients for embolectomy are carefully selected to include only those with large central emboli, then simple extraction of all *visible* central and distal clot will result in nearly complete normalization of pulmonary artery pressures. Leaving small, peripheral emboli behind is preferable to performing dangerous blind maneuvers to achieve a perfectly complete embolectomy. The pulmonary vasculature is known to possess a great capacity for fibrinolysis and is capable of clearing these peripheral emboli over time.

Weaning from Cardiopulmonary Bypass

The primary issue in weaning patients from cardiopulmonary bypass after embolectomy is right heart function. Although most patients will demonstrate immediate, often dramatic, improvements, some residual right ventricular stunning is common. Accurate right atrial and pulmonary artery pressures are critical and TEE is helpful. Volume loading and inotropic support may be necessary in the short term. Persistent elevation of pulmonary artery pressures must be investigated and treated expeditiously.

Inferior Vena Caval Filters

The role of inferior vena caval (IVC) filters in pulmonary embolectomy is controversial. About two-thirds of the reports advocate IVC interruption to avoid the uncommon, but often fatal, complication of early recurrent embolization. The alternative, early anticoagulation with heparin, does not completely eliminate the risk and may increase postoperative bleeding complications, particularly in patients with contraindications to thrombolytic therapy. The immediate postoperative period, before heparin can be safely initiated, may also be the period of greatest risk for reembolization. For these reasons, I believe most patients should undergo placement of an IVC filter. The low, but finite, incidence of filter complications (IVC thrombosis with recurrent embolization, migration, and chronic venous stasis) must, however, be considered, especially in younger patients in whom their cumulative incidence can be significant over a lifetime. We usually place the filter in the operating room just before sternal closure. It is advanced retrograde, through the right atrial appendage venous pursestring, into the infrarenal vena cava guided by a portable "C-arm" fluoroscope. Occasionally, a very stable patient who is already in the angiography suite for a pulmonary angiogram will undergo preoperative filter placement if the procedure can be completed with minimal delay.

Postoperative Management

Right heart function may take several days to normalize and aggressive support may be necessary during this period. Right atrial and pulmonary artery pressure, cardiac output, and mixed venous oxygen saturation should be carefully monitored. Strict attention to adequate ventilation and oxygenation is critical to avoid even transient pulmonary vasoconstriction. Inotropic agents should be weaned slowly. If a prolonged wean is anticipated, adding milrinone can permit catecholamines to be withdrawn. If an IVC filter has been placed, postoperative heparin therapy can be delayed for 24 to 48 h and started gently to maintain a partial thromboplastin time of 50 to 60 s. Warfarin can be initiated, with a target international normalized ratio (INR) of 2.0 to 2.5, once the patient is able to take oral medications. Long-term anticoagulation is usually continued for 6 months. A baseline echocardiogram and quantitative ventilation-perfusion scan are performed before discharge and repeated at 6 months to document resolution of any residual small perfusion defects and normalization of right heart function.

Summary

Surgical pulmonary embolectomy has a definite role to play in the management of selected patients with acute, major pulmonary embolism. Rapid noninvasive diagnostic modalities allow proper patient selection based on anatomic location of the emboli, right heart function, and contraindications to thrombolysis. Operative results are a direct reflection of the preoperative hemodynamic status, the degree of underlying cardiopulmonary disease, and attention to minimizing surgical trauma and protecting the right heart. An operative mortality of 10% or less and excellent long-term outcomes can be expected if the procedure is performed, before cardiovascular collapse, as part of a multidisciplinary strategy that emphasizes careful patient selection, rapid diagnosis, triage, and transport.

References

1. Goldhaber SZ, Visani L, De Rosa M. Acute pulmonary embolism: clinical outcomes in the International Cooperative Pulmonary Embolism Registry (ICOPER). Lancet 1999;353:1386–9.
2. Peterson KL. Acute pulmonary thromboembolism: has its evolution been redefined? Circulation 1999;99:1280–3.
3. Trendelenburg F. Uber die operative behandlung der embolie derlungarterie. Arch Klin Chir 1908;86:686–700.
4. Steenburg RW, Warren R, Wilson RE, et al. A new look at pulmonary embolectomy. Surg Gynecol Obstet 1958;107:214–20.
5. Romaine-Davis A. John Gibbon and his heart-lung machine. Philadelphia: University of Pennsylvania Press; 1991.
6. Allison PR, Dunhill MS, Marshall R. Pulmonary embolism. Thorax 1960;15:273–83.
7. Sautter RD, Lawron BR, Magnin GE. Pulmonary embolectomy: a simplified technique. Wis Med J 1962;61:309.
8. Cooley DA, Beall AC Jr, Alexander JK. Acute massive pulmonary embolism. Successful surgical treatment using temporary cardiopulmonary bypass. JAMA 1961;177:283–6.
9. Sharp EH. Pulmonary embolectomy: successful removal of a massive pulmonary embolus with support of cardiopulmonary bypass. Ann Surg 1962;156:1–4.
10. Kieny R, Charpentier A, Kieny MT. What is the place of pulmonary embolectomy today? J Cardiovasc Surg (Torino) 1991;32:549–54.
11. Clarke DB, Abrams LD. Pulmonary embolectomy: a 25 year experience. J Thorac Cardiovasc Surg 1986;92:442–5.
12. Stulz P, Schlapfer R, Feer R, et al. Decision making in the surgical treatment of massive pulmonary embolism. Eur J Cardiothorac Surg 1994;8:188–93.
13. Doerge H, Schoendube FA, Voss M, et al. Surgical therapy of fulminant pulmonary embolism: early and late results. Thorac Cardiovasc Surg 1999;47:9–13.
14. Ullmann M, Hemmer W, Hannekum A. The urgent pulmonary embolectomy: mechanical resuscitation in the operating theatre determines the outcome. Thorac Cardiovasc Surg 1999;47:5–8.
15. Doerge HC, Schoendube FA, Loeser H, et al. Pulmonary embolectomy: review of a 15-year experience and role in the age of thrombolytic therapy. Eur J Cardiothorac Surg 1996;10:952–7.
16. Jakob H, Vahl C, Lange R, et al. Modified surgical concept for fulminant pulmonary embolism. Eur J Cardiothorac Surg 1995;9:557–60; discussion 561.
17. Laas J, Schmid C, Albes JM, et al. Surgical aspects of fulminant pulmonary embolism. Z Kardiol 1993;82(suppl 2):25–8.
18. Meyns B, Sergeant P, Flameng W, et al. Surgery for massive pulmonary embolism. Acta Cardiol 1992;47:487–93.
19. Bauer EP, Laske A, von Segesser LK, et al. Early and late results after surgery for massive pulmonary embolism. Thorac Cardiovasc Surg 1991;39:353–6.
20. Schmid C, Zietlow S, Wagner TO, et al. Fulminant pulmonary embolism: symptoms, diagnostics, operative technique, and results. Ann Thorac Surg 1991;52:1102–5; discussion 1105–7.
21. Meyer G, Tamisier D, Sors H, et al. Pulmonary embolectomy: a 20-year experience at one center. Ann Thorac Surg 1991;51:232–6.
22. Morshuis WJ, van Son JA, Vincent JG, et al. Surgical treatment of massive pulmonary embolism. Ned Tijdschr Geneeskd 1990;134:1179–83.

23. Gray HH, Morgan JM, Paneth M, et al. Pulmonary embolectomy for acute massive pulmonary embolism: an analysis of 71 cases. Br Heart J 1988;60:196–200.
24. Glassford DM Jr, Alford WC Jr, Burrus GR, et al. Pulmonary embolectomy. Ann Thorac Surg 1981;32:28–32.
25. Tschirkov A, Krause E, Elert O, et al. Surgical management of massive pulmonary embolism. J Thorac Cardiovasc Surg 1978;75:730–3.
26. De Weese JA. The role of pulmonary embolectomy in venous thromboembolism. J Cardiovasc Surg (Torino) 1976;17:348–53.
27. Mattox KL, Feldtman RW, Beall AC Jr, et al. Pulmonary embolectomy for acute massive pulmonary embolism. Ann Surg 1982;195:726–31.
28. Shimokawa S, Watanabe S, Kobayashi A. Exsanguinating hemoptysis after pulmonary embolectomy. Ann Thorac Surg 1999;68:2385–6.
29. Wollman SB, Kushins LG. Survival following massive pulmonary hemorrhage complicating pulmonary embolectomy: a case report. Anesth Analg 1976;55:182–4.
30. Makey AR, Bliss BP, Ikram H, et al. Fatal intra-alveolar pulmonary bleeding complicating pulmonary embolectomy. Thorax 1971;26:466–71.
31. Habicht JM, Hammerli R, Perruchoud A, et al. Long-term follow-up in pulmonary embolectomy: is NYHA (dyspnea) classification reliable? Eur J Cardiothorac Surg 1996;10:32–7.
32. Soyer R, Brunet AP, Redonnet M, et al. Follow-up of surgically treated patients with massive pulmonary embolism–with reference to 12 operated patients. Thorac Cardiovasc Surg 1982;30:103–8.
33. Lund O, Nielsen TT, Ronne K, et al. Pulmonary embolism: long-term follow-up after treatment with full-dose heparin, streptokinase or embolectomy. Acta Med Scand 1987;221:61–71.
34. Heit JA, Mohr DN, Silverstein MD, et al. Predictors of recurrence after deep vein thrombosis and pulmonary embolism: a population-based cohort study. Arch Intern Med 2000;160:761–8.
35. Kasper W, Konstantinides S, Geibel A, et al. Management strategies and determinants of outcome in acute major pulmonary embolism: results of a multicenter registry. J Am Coll Cardiol 1997;30:1165–71.
36. Sasahara AA, Sharma GV, Barsamian EM, et al. Pulmonary thromboembolism. Diagnosis and treatment. JAMA 1983;249:2945–50.
37. Kasper W, Konstantinides S, Geibel A, et al. Prognostic significance of right ventricular afterload stress detected by echocardiography in patients with clinically suspected pulmonary embolism. Heart 1997;77:346–9.
38. Chapoutot L, Nazeyrollas P, Metz D, et al. Floating right heart thrombi and pulmonary embolism: diagnosis, outcome and therapeutic management. Cardiology 1996;87:169–74.
39. Casazza F, Bongarzoni A, Centonze F, et al. Prevalence and prognostic significance of right-sided cardiac mobile thrombi in acute massive pulmonary embolism. Am J Cardiol 1997;79:1433–5.
40. Chartier L, Bera J, Delomez M, et al. Free-floating thrombi in the right heart: diagnosis, management, and prognostic indexes in 38 consecutive patients. Circulation 1999;99:2779–83.
41. Goldhaber SZ. Optimal strategy for diagnosis and treatment of pulmonary embolism due to right atrial thrombus. Mayo Clin Proc 1988;63:1261–4.
42. Farfel Z, Shechter M, Vered Z, et al. Review of echocardiographically diagnosed right heart entrapment of pulmonary emboli-in-transit with emphasis on management. Am Heart J 1987;113:171–8.

43. Goldhaber SZ, Haire WD, Feldstein ML, et al. Alteplase versus heparin in acute pulmonary embolism: randomised trial assessing right-ventricular function and pulmonary perfusion. Lancet 1993;341:507–11.
44. Konstantinides S, Tiede N, Geibel A, et al. Comparison of alteplase versus heparin for resolution of major pulmonary embolism. Am J Cardiol 1998;82:966–70.
45. Konstantinides S, Geibel A, Olschewski M, et al. Association between thrombolytic treatment and the prognosis of hemodynamically stable patients with major pulmonary embolism: results of a multicenter registry. Circulation 1997;96:882–8.
46. Gulba DC, Schmid C, Borst HG, et al. Medical compared with surgical treatment for massive pulmonary embolism. Lancet 1994;343:576–7.
47. Jaumin P, Moriau M, el Gariani A, et al. Pulmonary embolectomy. Clinical experience. Acta Chir Belg 1986;86:123–5.
48. Stalpaert G, Suy R, Daenen W, et al. Surgical treatment of acute, massive lung embolism. Results and follow-up. Acta Chir Belg 1986;86:118–22.
49. Berger RL. Pulmonary embolectomy with preoperative circulatory support. Ann Thorac Surg 1973;16:217–27.
50. Heimbecker RO, Keon WJ, Richards KU. Massive pulmonary embolism. A new look at surgical management. Arch Surg 1973;107:740–6.
51. Aklog L, Williams CS, Byrne JG, et al. Acute pulmonary embolectomy—a contemporary approach. Circulation 2001;105:1416–9.

Catheter Interventions and Surgical Treatment of Pulmonary Embolism: Inferior Vena Cava Filter

Akihiro Niwa

Introduction

The inferior vena cava filter (IVCF) differs from anticoagulant therapy, fibrinolytic therapy, catheter intervention, emergency surgery, and other modes of treatment for acute pulmonary embolism (aPE) in that it does not address the thrombus itself in the pulmonary artery but is a medical device for the secondary prevention of thrombi in the acute stage.

A review of 34 consecutive cases of aPE clinically diagnosed between January 1985 and December 1995 shows that only 1 case (2.9%) died in the hospital in the acute phase but as many as 13 cases (32.8%) presented undeniable symptoms of aPE recurrence during hospitalization. Most of the aPE are caused by deep venous thrombosis (DVT). It is unlikely that all DVT disappear in the initial attack, and the presence of unstable and residual thrombi in the acute stage of aPE cannot be ignored. The acute stage of aPE can be safely managed by a reliable method of secondary prevention.

Residual Deep Venous Thrombosis After Acute Pulmonary Embolism

Girard et al. [1] conducted phlebography on 213 of 228 consecutive cases of aPE diagnosed by pulmonary arteriography and detected as many as 174 (81.7%) cases of DVT. They further reported that clinical symptoms or findings could be found in only 72 (41.2%) of those cases. In Japan as well, Hoshi et al. [2] conducted magnetic resonance imaging (MRI) on 28 aPE cases diagnosed by computed tomography (CT) and detected DVT in 26 (92.9%). These

Department of Cardiology, Musashino Red Cross Hospital, 1-26-1 Kyonan-cho, Musashino, Tokyo 180-8610, Japan

results suggest, therefore, that almost all aPE cases have residual DVT and that secondary prevention is an important issue in the management of acute-stage aPE patients.

Role of Inferior Vena Cava Filter in Acute Pulmonary Embolism Treatment

aPE usually becomes stable 1 to 2 weeks after the onset, and many patients can return to their activities of daily living (ADL). Basically, it is only in the early phase, when the patient's condition is still unstable, that the IVCF is needed. The IVCF is after all a foreign body and has inherent flaws, such as being an obstacle to catheter manipulation through the inferior vena cava and being a possible trigger of DVT in the chronic stage [3]. In light of these problems, a temporary filter (tIVCF) seems preferable to a permanent filter (pIVCF) in the treatment of aPE.

The requirements (Table 1) of a tIVCF that is clinically safe are as follows:

1. Has reliable capacity to capture thrombi
2. Does not damage the venous wall when the patient is mobile, because expanded ADL at an early stage is an important objective to prevent new DVT
3. Easy to manipulate, even in times of emergency
4. Enables intravenous drip of fluid from the tip of the IVCF to wash away microthrombi caused by inflammation of the venous wall
5. Can be used for several weeks
6. Easy to check for thrombi in the filter
7. Can be exchanged with a pIVCF when necessary

Retrievable filters have been developed in recent years, so these requirements will need to be revised in the future.

As of September 2003, there are six kinds of tIVCF commercially available in Japan (Fig. 1). In our hospital, we are using a Teflon filter called Neuhaus

TABLE 1. Requirement of temporary inferior vena cava (IVC) filter

Reliable capacity of capture of thrombosis
No damage to IVC wall without immobilization
Easy manipulation and management
Able to drip intravenously through the device
Able to use for a few weeks
Easy to check thrombus in the filter
Able to change to permanent IVC filter

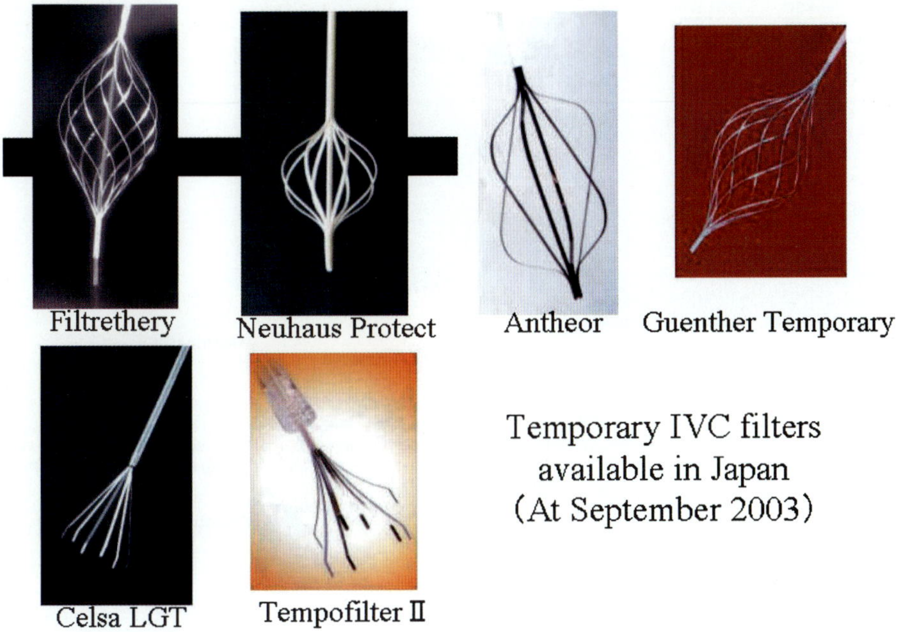

FIG. 1. Temporary inferior vena cava (*IVC*) filters available in Japan (as of September 2003)

Protect (Fig. 2) that enables intravenous drip from the tip and satisfies all the other conditions listed in Table 1. In experiments using simulated thrombi, when the diameter was larger than 7 mm the filter could capture all thrombi larger than 4 mm (Fig. 3). The results showed that the shorter the thrombi the lower the capture rate in thrombi less than 7 mm. In the clinical use of the IVCF we need to keep in mind the possibility of small thrombi escaping capture and finding their way to the pulmonary arteries.

Clinical Results After tIVCF Insertion

Subjects and Methods

The subjects were 99 cases who were diagnosed antemortem of 111 consecutive aPE cases managed in the acute stage at Musashino Red Cross Hospital from January 1985 to December 2002. Diagnosis was confirmed by pulmonary arteriography, contrast CT, lung perfusion scintigraphy, and echocardiogram. Treatment of aPE was mainly by anticoagulant and fibrinolytic therapy; no catheter treatment or emergency thrombectomy surgery was carried out.

We started to use the Neuhaus Protect in October 1996 and decided to use it in basically all acute-stage patients with the exception of those who did not

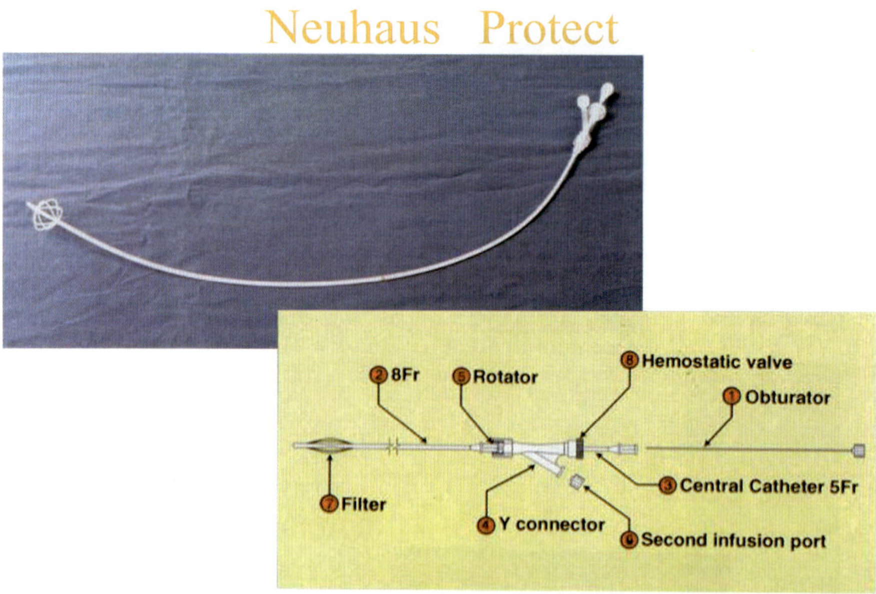

FIG. 2. Neuhaus Protect

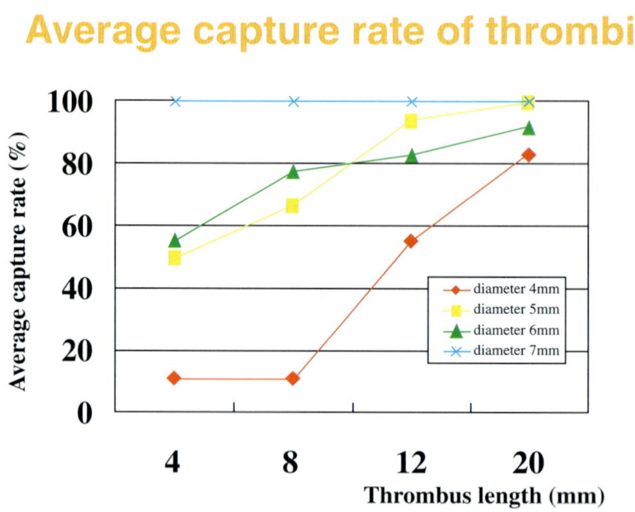

FIG. 3. Thrombus capture rate of Neuhaus Protect. Experiment tested the thrombus capture rate of Neuhaus Protect by passing simulated thrombi through a vertical steel pipe. At 7-mm diameter, all thrombi larger than 4 mm were captured. At smaller diameters, the capture rate declined

consent and those who could not be given drip infusion because of senility or other reasons. The subclavian vein was chosen as the site of puncture to facilitate early mobilization, and the patients were mobilized as soon as possible after their hemodynamics were stable. The case histories were studied retrospectively, and patients were divided into tIVCF use and nonuse for evaluation.

Results

There were 58 users and 41 nonusers of tIVCF. Backgrounds of the patients in both groups are shown in Table 2. There were no differences between the groups in the number of cancer cases, age, perioperative onset, critical cases, and deaths, but the in-hospital onset rate was high among the tIVCF users.

During management of the acute stage, cases who had new symptoms such as cough, chest pain, shortness of breath, wobbly gait, or restlessness were 6 of 58, or 10.3% among tIVCF users and 14 of 58 cases or 34.1%, a high percentage, among nonusers (Fig. 4). Deaths directly related to aPE occurred in 1 user and 2 nonusers. The tIVCF user mortality was a 53-year-old woman with a giant ovarian cancer who died of a relapse 14h after insertion of the tIVCF. Of the 2 nonuser mortalities, 1 was a patient with antiphospholipid antibody syndrome whose arteriovenous thrombus was resistant to treatment. The other was a patient who had cardiopulmonary arrest in the ambulance, came to the hospital in a state of shock, was diagnosed as aPE by echocardiography, and was given intra-aortic balloon pumping (IABP) and percutaneous cardiopulmonary support (PCPS) but did not respond. With regard to the complications of tIVCF (Table 3), there were 16 cases (27.5%) of

TABLE 2. Baseline characteristics of the patients

	Use of tIVCF	Nonuse of tIVCF
Case no.	58 patients	41 patients
Cancer no.	11 patients	8 patients
Male/female	19/39 patients	16/25 patients
Mean age	62.2 years old	65.3 years old
Setting period of tIVCF	2–26 days; mean 13.3 days	
tIVCF extraction	All 58 patients	
In-hospital onset	19 patients	6 patients
Perioperative onset	18 patients	10 patients
Critical case[a]	11 patients	13 patients
Death	6 patients	2 patients

tIVCF, temporary inferior vena cava filter

[a] Critical case: cardiopulmonary arrest/shock/syncope

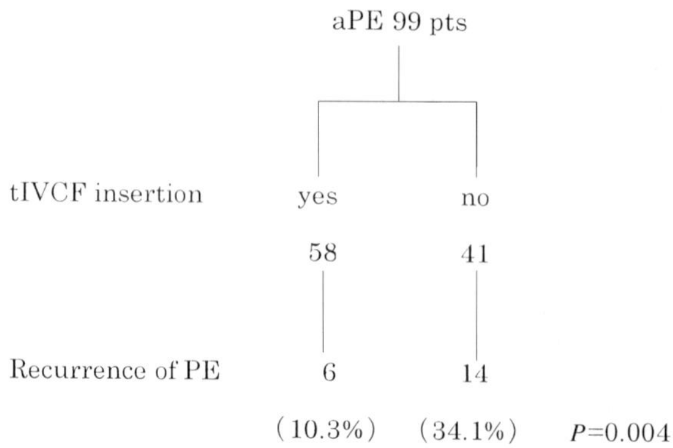

FIG. 4. Results of secondary prevention. Recurrence is defined by any symptoms (cough, chest pain, shortness of breath, etc.) during hospitalization. *aPE*, acute pulmonary embolism; *PE*, pulmonary embolism; *tIVCF*, temporary inferior vena cava filter

TABLE 3. Complications of temporary IVC filter

Bleeding/hematoma at puncture site: 16 (27.5%)
Thrombolysis for intrafilter thrombus: 7 (12.1%)
Slight fever: 6 (9.7%)
Retroperitoneal hematoma [percutaneous cardiopulmonary support (PCPS) site]: 1 (1.7%)
IVC occlusion: 1 (1.7%)
Filter migration: 1 (1.7%)
Pneumothorax: 0 (0%)

bleeding/hematoma at the puncture site. There were also 7 cases (12.1%) requiring thrombolysis for intrafilter thrombi, but in all cases the filter was removed after thrombolysis with no complications. Six cases had a slight fever of less than 38°C, which subsided in all cases after the tIVCF was removed. No cases of aerothorax were observed.

Transition to pIVCF was observed in 17 patients (29.3%) among the tIVCF users and in 12 patients among the nonusers, at the same rate of 29.3%. The reasons for using a permanent filter in the user group were poor ADL for 12, residual thrombi in the inferior vena cava for 3, inability to manage drug administration for 1, and 1 case of aPE after initial pIVCF insertion, managed by tIVCF during the acute phase and given pIVCF again after becoming stable. The reasons for using a permanent filter in the nonuser group were poor ADL for 3, aPE recurrence for 6, and anticoagulant therapy failure due to bleeding for 3.

Discussion

aPE may recur asymptomatically, and aPE recurrence has no specific symptoms. Even if any symptoms appear and are recorded by echocardiography, blood flow scintigraphy, CT, etc., similar records of the patient immediately before the events must be available for comparison to confirm that they are indeed symptoms of recurrence. That would be impossible, and there are many obstacles to obtaining an accurate recurrence rate. We therefore evaluated symptoms that appeared anew during acute-stage management of aPE which, although not perfect, are highly reliable indicators of aPE recurrence. The results suggested that tIVCF users present fewer new symptoms during use and are easier to control.

The tIVCF user who had a recurrence and died had a giant ovarian cancer with the tip of the tumor extending to the epigastrium. The inferior vena cava was extruded directly below the diaphragm by the tumor, and the tIVCF had to be placed inside the flattened inferior vena cava. When the Neuhaus Protect, which is made of Teflon, is dilated inside a flattened inferior vena cava it is easily distorted, so its ability to capture thrombi must have been compromised. On the other hand, we thought it was highly probable that a metallic tIVCF would injure the vascular wall and decided against it. Secondary prevention in cases like this is considered to be an important issue for the future.

The most frequent complication of tIVCF was bleeding/hematoma of the puncture site. Because the basic treatments for aPE are anticoagulant therapy and fibrinolytic therapy [4], and the shaft of the tIVCF is extracorporeal, caution is constantly required to prevent this complication. The best way to prevent it is to improve the attending clinician's technique and to puncture the vein at the first attempt. The complications that are generally cited in connection with tIVCF use are hemorrhagic complications caused by basic aPE therapy [5], filter displacement, venous thrombus, infections, air embolism, and filter breakage. Thrombus in the filter site is another complication [6] that should be considered. When contrast radiography of the filter site at the time of removal revealed a thrombus occupying more than one-fourth of the lumen, we administered fibrinolytic treatment from the filter tip. The thrombus size was reduced in all cases, and the filter could be removed in a few days without any problems.

The major reason for using a pIVCF was poor ADL in the tIVCF users and APE recurrence in the nonusers. ADL is determined by the underlying disease condition and poor ADL is a major risk factor for DVT, so the use of pIVCF was inevitable in such cases. pIVCF use due to aPE recurrence could be avoided by using tIVCF, which is considered to be clinically effective in acute-stage control.

The basic principle of aPE prevention is extended ADL. Long-term bed rest slows the venous blood flow rate and encourages the formation of venous thrombi, so it should be avoided as much as possible. Although recurrence could easily occur when shifting from bed rest to expanded ADL, we believe that if unstable DVT entering the venous bloodstream are captured by the tIVCF, expanded ADL can proceed safely in the acute phase.

As retrievable filters that can be removed with certainty are developed in the future, we can look forward to fewer complications of bleeding and infections and the realization of aPE acute-stage management that is safer than ever before.

Summary

Use of tIVCF in aPE was effective in the stabilization of symptoms and management of the acute stage. When using the tIVCF, however, one needs to guard against bleeding at the puncture site and infection and consider measures against intrafilter thrombi.

References

1. Girard P, Musset D, Parent F, et al. High prevalence of detectable deep venous thrombosis in patients with acute pulmonary embolism. Chest 1999;116:903–8.
2. Hoshi T, Hachiya T. Evaluation of embolic source of pulmonary thromboembolism using lower limb MR venography. Jpn J Phlebot 2002;13(4):267–72 (English abstract).
3. Decousus H, Leizorovicz A, Parent F, et al. A clinical trial of vena caval filters in the prevention of pulmonary embolism in patients with proximal deep-vein thrombosis: Prevention du Risque d'Embolie Pulmonaire par Interruption Cave Study Group. N Engl J Med 1998;338(7):409–15.
4. Task Force Report. Guidelines on diagnosis and management of acute pulmonary embolism. Eur Heart J 2000;21:1301–36.
5. Zwaan VM, Kagel C, Marienhoff N, et al. Erste Erfahrungen mit temporaeren Vena-cava-Filtern. Fortschr Roentgenstr 1995;163(2):171–6.
6. Lorch H, Welger D, Wagner V, et al. Current practice of temporary vana cava filter insertion: a multicenter registry. J Vasc Interv Radiol 200;11(1):83–8.

3. Traveler's Thrombosis

Pulmonary Thromboembolism Associated with Air Travel in Japan

Hiroshi Morio

Introduction

Recently the link between venous thromboembolism (VTE) and air travel has been discussed [1, 2]. The first report of deep-vein thrombosis associated with air travel was published in 1954 [3]. In 1977, three cases of acute pulmonary thromboembolism (PTE) after air travel were reported and called economy class syndrome [4]. Since the 1980s, many cases of acute PTE after air travel have been reported and called economy class syndrome [5], coach class thrombosis [6], or traveler's thrombosis [7] in Europe and the United States.

In Japan, the first report of acute PTE associated with air travel was published in 1996 [8], and only 45 cases of acute PTE after air travel have been reported. Our hospital is the closest general hospital to Narita Airport (New Tokyo International Airport), and 24 cases were admitted to our hospital from 1994 to 2002. Our cases were half of all cases of acute PTE associated with air travel in Japan, so our data may represent acute PTE after air travel in Japan.

The purpose of this study is to clarify the characteristics of acute PTE associated with air travel in Japan.

Patients and Methods

Patients

Twenty-four patients hospitalized in our hospital for acute PTE associated with air travel from 1994 to 2002 were investigated. During this period, 49 patients with acute PTE were hospitalized in our hospital, so patients with

Department of Internal Medicine, Narita Red Cross Hospital, 90-1 Iida-cho, Narita, Chiba 286-8523, Japan

acute PTE associated with air travel were 49% (24/49) of all patients with acute PTE.

Methods

The study design was retrospective. For patient characteristics, nationality, age, sex, height, body weight, and risk factors for PTE were investigated. Risk factors for PTE are classified to low risk, moderate risk, or high risk as follows: low risk: obesity, active inflammation, hyperlipidemia, diabetes, smoking, and recent minor surgery (within last 3 days); moderate risk: varicose veins, heart failure (uncontrolled), recent myocardial infarction (within 6 weeks), hormone therapy (including oral contraception), pregnancy/postpartum, lower limb paralysis, intravenous catheter, or lower limb trauma (within 6 weeks); and high risk: previous VTE, family history of VTE, known thrombophilia, previous cerebral vascular attack (CVA), malignancy, or recent major surgery (within 6 weeks). A coagulation search for prothrombin time, APTT, antithrombin III, protein S, protein C, lupus anticoagulant, and anticardiolipin antibody was made. For travel information, duration of flight, class and position of seats, and times which patients left their seats flight were investigated.

Results

Patient Characteristics

One case was from Chinese Taipei, and the other 23 cases were Japanese. Only 2 cases were male; the other 22 cases were female. They were from 39 to 75 years old (60.0 ± 9.8 years, mean ± SD). Most of the cases were over 40 years of age. They were from 147 to 160 cm tall (157.0 ± 6.5 cm); two-thirds of the patients were under 160 cm. Their body weight ranged from 49 to 77 kg (59.5 ± 8.5 kg). Body mass index (BMI) of the patients was from 20.7 to 32.0 (24.1 ± 2.7 kg/m^2). Obese cases, whose BMI was over 25, comprised only 4 cases. Fifteen cases had risk factors for VTE; 7 cases of varicose vein, 6 cases of hyperlipidemia, 4 cases of obesity, 2 cases of malignancy or history of PTE, and 1 case of smoking or contraceptive. On the other hand, 9 cases, one-third of all cases, had no risk factors for VTE.

Table 1 shows comparison of risk factors of PTE with or without air travel. The air travel group was 24 cases and the group without air travel was 25 cases. Fifteen cases of PTE in the group with air travel had risk factors (4 cases of low risk, 7 cases of moderate risk, and 4 cases of high risk). In PTE without air travel, 23 cases had risk factors (5 cases of low risk, 5 cases of moderate risk, and 13 cases of high risk). No cases had coagulation abnormalities in either group. Idiopathic PTE, that is, PTE without risk factor and coagulation abnormalities, constituted 9 cases; 38% in PTE were in the group with air travel. Idiopathic PTE were significantly more common in PTE in the group

TABLE 1. Comparison of risk factors in pulmonary thromboembolism (PTE) with or without air travel

	PTE with air travel group ($n = 24$)	PTE without air travel group ($n = 25$)	P value (χ^2 test)
Low risk	4	5	NS
Moderate risk	7	5	NS
High risk	4	13	0.010
Positive for coagulation search	0	0	NS
Idiopathic PTE	9	2	0.015

NS, not significant

with air travel than in the group without air travel. Moreover, cases with high risk were significantly fewer in PTE in the group with air travel than in the group without air travel.

All cases flew more than 8h, and duration of flight was from 8 to 14h (11.4 ± 1.9h, mean ± SD). Ten cases flew from the United States mainland, 4 cases from Hawaii, 9 cases from Europe, and 1 case from Australia. There was no case from Asia.

Only 1 case flew in business class, and the other 23 cases were in economy class. Eight cases were in window seats, 10 cases were in inside seats, and 5 cases were on aisle seats (seat position for 1 case was unknown). Cases in window or inside seats were more common than in aisle seats. In the plane, there are about the same numbers of inside seats as aisle seats, but numbers of window seats are half of inside or aisle seats. So, PTE occurred more often in patients in window or inside seats than in patients in aisle seats.

Seventeen cases, two-thirds of all cases, did not leave their seats at all. They remained sitting for a long time during the flight. Time leaving seats during flight was 0.5 ± 0.9, mean ± SD.

The most common symptoms were dyspnea and syncope (17 cases for each symptom). Syncope is the symptom of severe cases, so many cases in this study were severe cases.

Clinical Course

Anticoagulation therapy by heparin, and thrombolytic therapy by urokinase or tissue plasminogen activator (t-PA) was given to the patients. A permanent inferior vena cava (IVC) filter was inserted into 1 patient with recurrent PTE. One patient had intrafemoral hemorrhage, which was the side effect of thrombolytic therapy. There was 1 case associated with cerebral infarction. This case is shown in the following case report. Duration of stay in the hospital was from 10 to 39 days (18.3 ± 6.8 days, mean ± SD). Fortunately, all 24 cases recovered to be discharged.

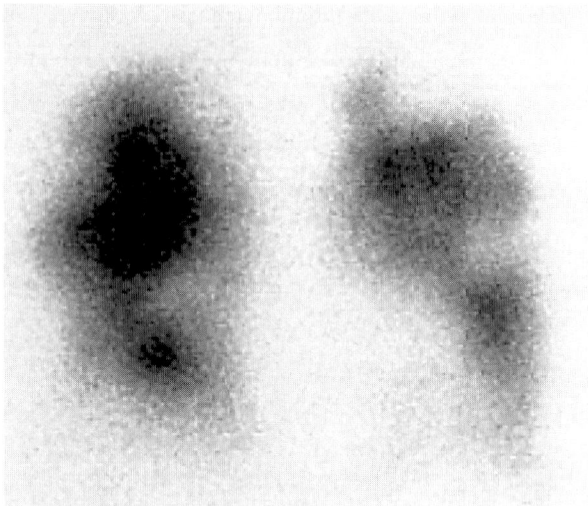

FIG. 1. Lung perfusion scan (4th day)

Case Report

A 75-year-old woman flew from Rome to Narita in economy class seat for 14h. Soon after she departed from the plane, she felt motor and sensory disturbance in her left side and she had syncope for some minutes. She was taken by ambulance to our hospital. On admission, she showed clear consciousness, normal blood pressure (142/79 mmHg), and left hemiparesis. She showed low oxygen concentration (PaO_2, 68.6 torr). Although computed tomography (CT) scan on the first and second days showed normal findings, the diagnosis of cerebral infarction was made for her symptoms. She was treated with sodium ozagrel and ticlopidine. Her hemiparesis and sensory disturbance were fully recovered on the second day. Lung perfusion scan on the 4th day showed multiple perfusion defects in both lungs, suggesting pulmonary thromboembolism (Fig. 1). Echocardiography (TTE) on the seventh day showed normal findings; the foramen ovale was not patent. MRI on the ninth day (Fig. 2) showed a small infarction in the right putamen and parietal lobe, suggesting lacunar infarction. Pulmonary angiography on the tenth day showed normal findings, suggesting that the thrombi in her pulmonary artery disappeared following thrombolytic therapy.

Discussion

Recently the link between VTE and air travel has been discussed [1, 2]. Since the 1980s, many cases of acute PTE after air travel have been reported in Europe and the United States [3, 7]. On the other hand, only 45 cases of acute

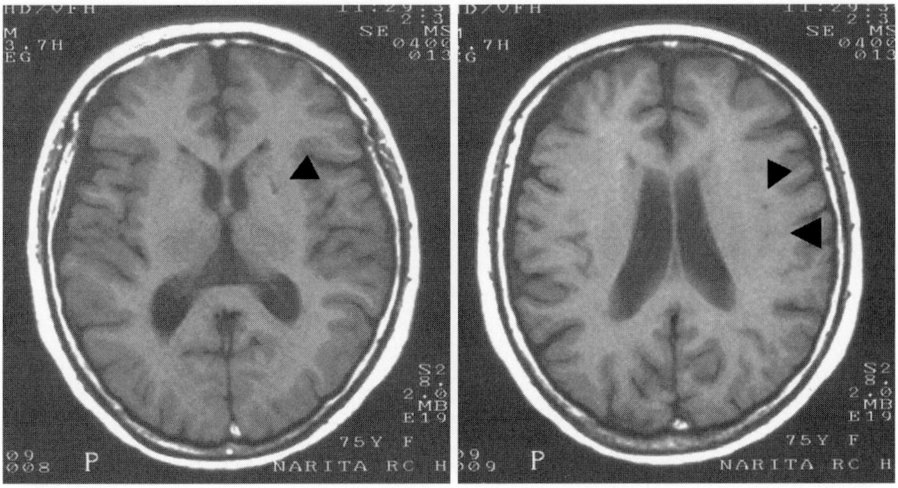

FIG. 2. Magnetic resonance imaging (MRI) findings (T1 image, 9th day). *Arrowheads*, low density area suggesting infarction

PTE after air travel have been reported in Japan. In this article, we showed 24 cases of acute PTE after air travel. Our cases were half of all cases of acute PTE associated with air travel in Japan. Table 2 shows all cases of acute PTE after air travel reported in Japan. Most of the reports were case reports. Details of patient characteristics were not shown in many reports. Total data for age, sex, flight time, and risks were almost the same as our data. Our data may represent acute PTE after air travel in Japan.

In Japan, acute PTE associated with air travel occurred in short persons more frequently than in tall persons. Figure 3 shows a hypothesis of the reason PTE occurs more frequently in short persons [5]. A short person has short legs, and has a small space between their legs and the seat. Pressure on the calves from the edge of the seat, possibly more common in a short person, will exacerbate venous stasis.

Acute PTE associated with air travel occurred in women more frequently than in men in Japan. There are two possible reasons. First, in Japan, most women are short. Second, Japanese women may be too shy to walk to the washroom if they take a window or inside seat.

In this study, idiopathic PTE, that is, PTE without risk factors and coagulation abnormalities, occurred significantly more often in the air travel group than in the group without air travel. Moreover, cases with high risk were significantly fewer in the group of PTE with air travel than the group without air travel. These data suggest that air travel itself may be a risk factor for PTE.

We had one case of acute PTE associated with cerebral infarction after air travel. Recently, Lapostolle et al. reported cases of cerebral infarction associ-

Table 2. Acute PTE after air travel reported in Japan

Author	Year	No. of cases	Age (years)	Sex	Flight time (h)	Seat	Risk
Yamashita	1996	1	53	M	13.5	U	+
Satoh	1996	1	52	F	9.5	E	–
Yokoyama	2000	1	69	F	12.4	U	–
Rhujin	2001	1	72	F	10.0	U	–
Kuwano	2001	3	43, 59, 82	F3	11.7, 11.8, 13.7	E3	+2/–1
Katada	2001	1	69	F	13.0	U	–
Hirano	2001	1	28	M	20.0	U	–
Furumatsu	2002	1	65	M	U	U	+
Morimoto	2002	1	66	F	12	U	+
Hata	2002	10	61 ± 9	M1/F9	15 (mean)	U	U
Our data	2003	24	60.0 ± 9.8	M2/F22	11.4 ± 1.9	E23/B1	+15/–9
Total		45	59.9 ± 11.5	M6/F39	11.8 ± 2.3	E27/B1	+20/–15

M, male; F, female; U, unknown; E, economy class; B, business class

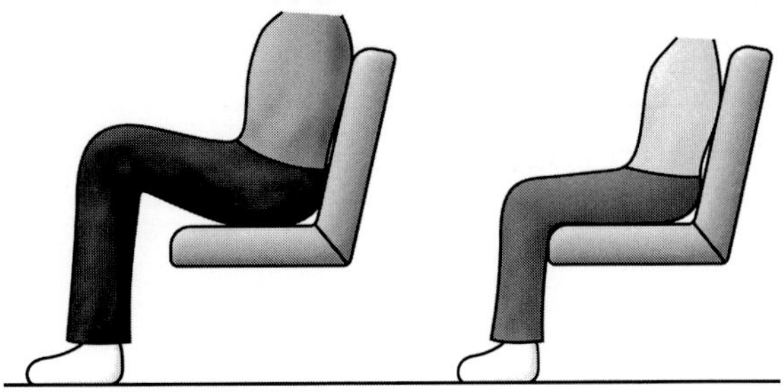

FIG. 3. Hypothesis of the reason why pulmonary thromboembolism (PTE) occurs in short persons more frequently than in tall persons

ated with pulmonary embolism after air travel [9]. They suggested a patent foramen ovale played an important role in paradoxical embolism. In our case, the foramen ovale was not patent, and the magnetic resonance imaging (MRI) finding did not suggest paradoxical embolism, but lacunar infarction. Her symptoms were recovered rapidly. It is supposed that she had an old infarction, and transient decreased blood pressure or low oxygen concentration caused by PTE induced her symptoms.

In conclusion, acute PTE associated with air travel in Japan tended to occur in elderly people, females, and short people. It tended to occur in occupants of window seats and inside seats more frequently than in those in aisle seats. Most of the patients did not leave their seats during flights. In common cases, PTE occurred immediately after starting to walk after long-haul flights.

References

1. Gallus AS, Goghlan DC. Travel and venous thrombosis. Curr Opin Pulmon Med 2002;8:372–8.
2. O'Keeffe DJ, Baglin TP. Traveller's thrombosis and economy class syndrome: incidence, aetiology and prevention. Clin Lab Haemost 2003;25:277–81.
3. Homans J. Thrombosis of the deep leg veins due to prolonged sitting. N Engl J Med 1954;250:148–9.
4. Symington IS, Stack BHR. Pulmonary thromboembolism after travel. Br J Dis Chest 1977;71:138–40.
5. Cruickshank JM, Gorlin R, Jennett B. Air travel and thrombotic episodes: The economy class syndrome. Lancet 1988;ii:497–8.
6. Arfvidsson B, Eklof B, Kistner RL, et al. Risk factors for venous thromboembolism following prolonged air travel: coach class thrombosis. Haematol Oncol Clin N Am 2000;14:391–400.
7. Bagshaw M. Traveller's thrombosis: a review of deep vein thrombosis associated with travel. Aviat Space Environ Med 2001;72:848–51.
8. Yamashita M, Mori Y ,Shimada T, et al. A case of economy class syndrome (in Japanese). Rinsyo-Kakuigaku 1996;29:105–7.
9. Lapostolle F, Borron SW, Surget V, et al. Stroke associated with pulmonary embolism after air travel. Neurology 2003;60:1983–5.

Thromboembolic Events Associated with Air Travel

F. Lapostolle, J. Catineau, and F. Adnet

French Emergency Medical System

In France, out-of-hospital medical emergencies are managed by the Service d'Aide Médicale Urgente (SAMU) [1]. There is a nationwide phone number to contact the regional emergency physician dispatcher of the SAMU, 24h per day. The dispatcher can transfer the request to other services (fire or police departments, for example) in cases of nonmedical emergencies. In contrast, in cases of medical emergencies, the dispatcher can give telephonic assistance, or send on site a light ambulance, a general practitioner, or a mobile intensive care unit. In each mobile intensive care unit ambulance, the squad is composed of a trained driver, an emergency nurse, and an experienced emergency physician. Ambulances on emergency standby (seven in our hospital and others within the region) can be sent on site by the dispatcher, who is receiving calls from a suburban area of Paris that has a population of 1.5 million habitants. SAMU and the emergency dispatcher are also responsible for transfer from medical units and interhospital transfers when patients require intensive care. This is the reason why for many years we have been interested in patients with pulmonary embolism transferred from Roissy-Charles-de Gaulle Airport to different hospitals.

Relation Between Air Travel and Thromboembolic Events

The recent history of the relation between travel and thromboembolic events should be summarized with three dates: 1954, when Homans reported 5 cases of patients with thromboembolic events, including deep venous thrombosis

SAMU 93, UPRES 34-09, Hôpital Avicenne, 125, Rue de Stalingrad, 93009, Bobigny, France

after prolonged air travel [2]; 1967, when Beighton reported the first pulmonary embolism after air travel [3]; and 1977, when Symington proposed the "economy class syndrome" term for these events [4]. In a study of 182 patients with pulmonary embolism, 3 patients reported recent prolonged air travel in economy class. Conditions of travel in economy class were supposed to decrease mobility and to be responsible for an increased thromboembolic events incidence. Roughly 100 cases of pulmonary embolism occurring after air travel have been published during the last three decades. Most of these reports have included limited numbers of patients, combined deep venous thrombosis and pulmonary embolism, or included poorly documented cases. Thus, although the number of passengers continues to increase, the relationship between pulmonary embolism and air travel remained strongly disputed.

The three factors of Virchow's triad [5], that is, venous stasis, vessel wall injury, and hypercoagulability, appear to be present during air travel, increasing the risk of venous thrombosis development. The sitting position is associated with venous stasis, a significant decrease in blood flow, an increase in hematocrit, and in blood protein concentration in the legs after only 1 h [6, 7]. Immobility increases thrombi formation. Landgraf and colleagues simulated a flight of 12 h and demonstrated that blood viscosity increased in relation with patients' immobility. Finally, vessel lesions due to the compression by the seat have been advocated [6]. Conditions are present to increase thromboembolic events during air travel but, in contrast, the relation between prolonged air travel and thromboembolism events remained disputed [8–10].

We thus chose to undertake a more objective evaluation of this association [11]. The aim of our study was to test the hypothesis that duration of air travel was a risk factor for pulmonary embolism. To do so, we systematically reviewed all documented cases of pulmonary embolism requiring medical care upon arrival at Roissy-Charles-de-Gaulle Airport, France's busiest international airport.

Prospective Study

Inclusion Criteria

All patients arriving at Roissy Charles de Gaulle (CDG) Airport requiring medical care and transport to hospital by a French prehospital medical team (SAMU 93) for suspected pulmonary embolism were systematically reviewed. It should be noted that SAMU is responsible for all patients requiring emergency transport from CDG. Suspicion of pulmonary embolism was based on the occurrence of clinical criteria within 1 h of arrival at CDG Airport. Clinical criteria suggesting pulmonary embolism included chest pain, malaise, syncope, or shortness of breath. Final diagnosis of pulmonary embolism was confirmed by high-probability scintigraphic ventilation-perfusion scan, pulmonary angiography, or high-resolution helical computed tomographic angiography. Patients in whom the diagnosis of pulmonary embolism was subsequently ruled out were excluded. The period of inclusion was from November 1993 to December 2000.

Roissy-Charles-de-Gaulle Airport Data

A list of all passengers arriving at CDG Airport, year by year, with the initial geographical origins of all flights, numbers of passengers, by country, distance, and duration of air travel were obtained from the Aéroports de Paris (ADP) to evaluate the incidence rates.

Patient Data

For all patients included in this study, the following data were obtained: initial origin of the flight by country, distance, duration, and class of travel. Physical activity during the flight, defined as walking in the plane, was recorded at the patient interview by the physician of SAMU 93. General risk factors for thromboembolic events were classified as high or moderate risk factors (Table 1).

The elements of the clinical presentation were documented, including time of onset of the first symptom [during the flight, on standing up after landing, on exiting the plane (i.e., in the jetway), or in the airport], the occurrence of cardiac arrest, chest pain, malaise, and dyspnea. Results of scintigraphic ventilation-perfusion scan, angiography, or high-resolution helical computed tomographic angiography were recorded.

Severity of pulmonary embolism was assessed according to published criteria: syncope, clinically apparent acute right ventricular dysfunction, shock [defined as *systolic arterial pressure* (SAP) less than 80 mm Hg], tachycardia [defined as *pulse rate* (PR) more than 120 bpm], and angiographic Miller

TABLE 1. Risk factors for thromboembolic events

High risk factors	Moderate risk factors
Recent immobilization (greater than 3 days)	Varicose veins
Recent surgery	Oral contraceptive use
Multiple trauma (less than 3 weeks prior)	Hormonal replacement therapy
Previous deep venous thrombosis	Age greater than 40 years
Previous pulmonary embolism	Obesity
Known malignant disease	Tobacco use
Current pregnancy or immediate postpartum period	Nephrotic syndrome
History of congestive heart failure	
Coagulation disorders	

index (defined as an obstruction of greater than 50% of the pulmonary arterial bed). Duration of stay in the hospital and final outcomee were recorded.

Statistical Analysis

Results are expressed as mean ± SD. Quantitative parameters were compared using a two-tailed Student's *t* test and qualitative parameters using the chi-squared test, with $P < 0.05$ arbitrarily chosen as significant. The incidence of pulmonary embolism as a function of distance traveled was calculated in cases per million passenger arrivals in increments of 2500 km.

Results

Patient Data

Fifty-six patients with confirmed pulmonary embolism were included. Forty-two patients (75%) were female and 14 (25%) were male. The mean age was 57 ± 12 years, without significant difference between males and females.

The origin of these patients is reported in Fig. 1. The incidence of pulmonary embolism, expressed as number of cases per million passengers per 2500 km traveled, increased with the distance traveled (Fig. 2). The risk of pulmonary embolism significantly increased after 5000 km ($P < 10^{-4}$). The total incidence of pulmonary embolism reached 4.8 cases per million passengers for travels of greater than 7500 km. Pulmonary embolism incidence

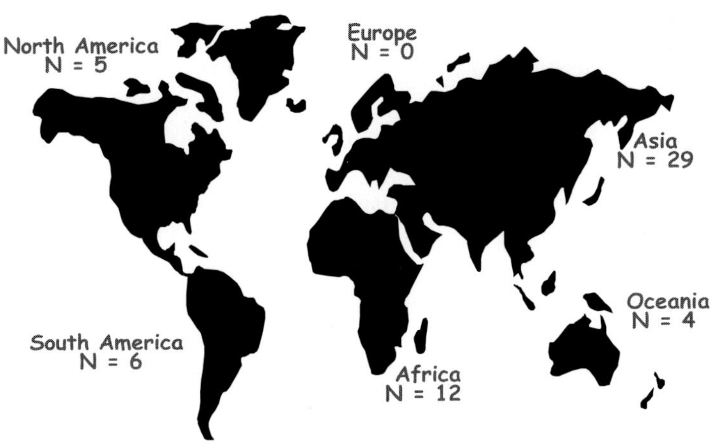

FIG. 1. Origin of passengers with pulmonary embolism arriving at Reissy-Charles-de-Gaulle-Airport (France)

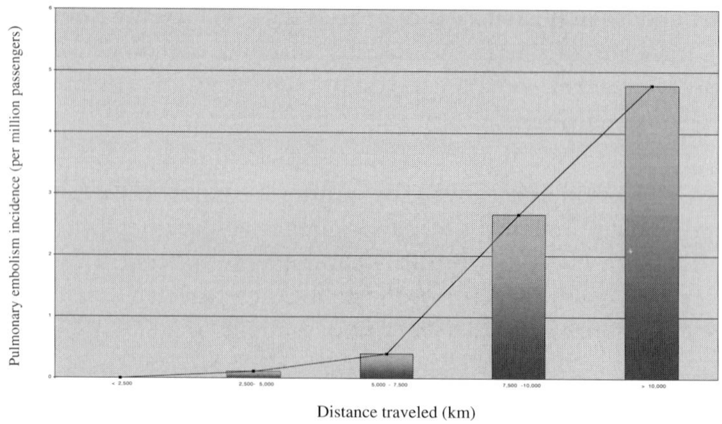

FIG. 2. Incidence of pulmonary embolism according to distance traveled. (From [11], with permission)

increased by a factor of 11 for travels of more than 5000 km in comparison with travels of less than 5000 km.

Travel occurred in economy (tourist) class in 42 cases (75%) and in business class in 2 cases (4%). These data were unavailable in 12 cases (21%). Physical activity (walking) during air travel was reported in only 3 cases (5%) and complete immobility in 42 cases (75%). These data were unavailable in 11 cases (20%). High and moderate risk factors for thromboembolic diseases were reported in 4 (7%) and 49 patients (87%), respectively.

The first symptom suggesting pulmonary embolism occurred during air travel in 8 cases (14%), upon standing after landing in 16 cases (29%), and in the jetway in 32 cases (57%). In no case did the primary manifestation occur beyond the jetway, that is, inside the airport. The first symptom was malaise in 54 cases (96%) associated with syncope in half of these (48%), dyspnea in 36 cases (64%), and chest pain in 20 cases (36%). At the time of the first (on-site) medical examination, one patient presented in cardiac arrest and was successfully resuscitated.

Diagnosis of pulmonary embolism was confirmed by high-probability scintigraphic ventilation-perfusion scan in 21 cases (37%), angiography in 9 cases (16%), and high-resolution helical computed tomographic angiography in 16 cases (29%). In 40 cases (25%) more than one examination was performed. Emboli were bilateral in 53 cases (95%). In the 9 cases where angiography was performed, the Miller index was superior to 50% in 7 cases. Transthoracic echocardiography was performed in 25 cases (45%), with acute right ventricular dysfunction reported in 17 cases.

At least one criterion for severe pulmonary embolism was found in each patient: syncope in 27 cases (48%), acute right ventricular dysfunction in 30 cases (54%), shock in 6 cases (11%), tachycardia in 15 cases (27%), Miller index greater than 50% in 9 cases (16%), and cardiac arrest in 1 case (2%).

The mean duration of hospital stay was 7 ± 4 days. One patient, whose pulmonary embolism was complicated by an ischemic cerebral stroke due to paradoxical embolism, died.

Stroke as a Particular Clinical Presentation

During an 8-year period (from 1993 to 2001), among 65 patients with pulmonary embolism, 4 were diagnosed with thromboembolic stroke, defined as focal neurological deficit(s) associated with acute ischemic infarct on CT scan. Transesophageal contrast echocardiography revealed a patent foramen ovale in each case [12]. We undertook a descriptive study of such unusual clinical presentations of patients with pulmonary embolism after air travel (Table 2).

Stroke caused by paradoxical embolism as a complication of severe pulmonary embolism was an unusual thromboembolic event after prolonged air travel, in our study. This incidence may be underestimated because patients who died for any reason, including severe cerebral infarction and pulmonary embolism, were not included, and because pulmonary embolism may have gone undiagnosed among patients whose principal clinical presentation was characterized by neurological impairment. Stroke after air travel has been reported in the absence of deep venous thrombosis or pulmonary embolism [12, 13]. However, the relation between stroke without pulmonary embolism and air travel has never been demonstrated, allowing one to imagine that such an event during air travel might occur by chance alone.

TABLE 2. Characteristic of four patients with stroke and pulmonary embolism after air travel

Case 1	Case 2	Case 3	Case 4
53-year-old woman	67-year-old woman	51-year-old woman	56-year-old man
Los Angeles–Paris 9080 km, 10.5 h	Rio de Janeiro–Paris 9170 km, 11 h	Phnom Penh–Paris 9450 km, 11.25 h	New York–Paris 5840 km, 8 h
In the jetway	In the plane, before landing	In the plane, before landing	In the plane, before landing
Conscious impairment, complete left hemiplegia, left facial paralysis	Conscious impairment, right hemiparesis, aphasia	Coma, left hemiplegia	Coma, right hemiplegia, aphasia
Five months later, persistent hemiparesis	Two months later, persistent aphasia	Death on day 3	Nine months later, persistent hemiplegia and aphasia

Patent foramen ovale is known to be associated with a poor prognosis in patients with pulmonary embolism [14]. In our recent study including 56 patients with severe pulmonary embolism, the lone patient who died suffered both pulmonary embolism and stroke (case 3) [11]. The remaining patients of the present study had persistent neurological deficit.

Finally, it should be noted that interactions between these two pathologies are important. One of the diagnoses, stroke or pulmonary embolism, might be missed and treatment of the patient with concomitant pulmonary embolism and stroke poses special risks; first, because thrombolysis and anticoagulant therapy may aggravate brain injuries and conversely because when neurological injury dominates the clinical presentation, undiagnosed pulmonary embolism may be responsible for additional thromboembolic events and aggravation of cerebral hypoxia.

Discussion

The relation between duration of air travel and pulmonary embolism is clearly established in this study. The incidence of pulmonary embolism increased dramatically for travel of more than 5000 km or approximately 6 h of flight duration, demonstrating that distance is a significant risk factor for pulmonary embolism. All patients with pulmonary embolism had traveled at least 4000 km. The increased incidence of pulmonary embolism with increased travel duration was not due to an increased duration of the "observation" period alone. If this were the case, the increase would be expected to be constant.

We strongly believe that the incidence of pulmonary embolism was underestimated in our study, first, because patients with cardiac arrest during flight, after landing, or in the airport were not included in this study. The percentage of cardiac arrests occurring in flight or immediately after landing that might be attributable to pulmonary embolism is unknown. Furthermore, deaths pronounced as being due to pulmonary embolism occurring before care was performed by the prehospital medical team (SAMU 93) were probably responsible for the low mortality rate reported in this study. The second reason was failure to detect less-severe cases. Severe pulmonary embolism represents approximately 20% of clinical presentations of pulmonary embolism; thus, one might expect an incidence of pulmonary embolism after flights of more than 7500 km of approximately 25 per million passengers. In our study, only the presence of severe clinical signs, in particular, syncope, resulted in a call for emergency medical services. It is probable that passengers with minor signs, such as mild to moderate chest pain, fever, or calf pain, leave the airport without medical consultation and thus without a diagnosis.

Several reports have suggested that passengers may develop pulmonary embolism several weeks after air travel [16, 17]. In the same way, we speculate that the incidence of deep venous thrombosis is likely high after long-distance air travel. In the Lonflit studies, such events were reported in almost 5% of the patients [18, 19].

Other Risk Factors

The duration of flight appears as a major contributing risk factor for severe pulmonary embolism associated with travel, as "long distance air travel syndrome." The role of other risk factors is still unknown, which is problematic to optimize prophylactic treatment. In our study, only four patients had factors generally agreed to be of high risk for pulmonary embolism. Most of them had moderate risk factors. Unfortunately, our methodology does not permit us to discern the importance of risk factors other than duration of flight (as the denominators are unknown) including nature of travel class and immobility. To identify other risk factors, we studied the sex ratio. In effect, our study included 93 patients (1993–2002), with 72% being women. Such sex repartition is unusual in pulmonary embolism studies. Then, female sex could be an independent risk factors. Due to the rarity of thromboembolic events, it is illusive to undergo prospective study to test this hypothesis. Then, using Bayes theorem, postulating that the sex ratio in flight was 1 : 1, we calculated pulmonary embolism for men and women. The probability was 2.2 for 1 million passengers for men and 1.6 for women. To determine optimal prophylactic treatment, such calculation should be performed for each potential risk factor. The difficulty is that the prevalence of each factor in travelers is currently unknown.

Conclusions

The duration of flight appears as a major contributing risk factor for severe pulmonary embolism associated with travel. Given the risk of air travel of long duration, behavioral, mechanical, and pharmacological prophylactic measures should be considered. Behavioral and mechanical prophylactic measures are easy to perform and include abundant consumption of non-alcoholic beverages, refraining from smoking, avoidance of tight clothing that may limit blood flow, use of elastic support stockings, avoidance of leg-crossing, frequent changes of position while seated, and minor physical activity, such as walking, or at least moving the limbs. These measures and, perhaps, pharmacological measures, are insufficiently documented to suggest precise indications.

References

1. Nikkanen HE, Pouges C, Jacobs LM. Emergency medicine in France. Ann Emerg Med 1998;31:116–20.
2. Homans J. Thrombosis of the leg veins due to prolonged sitting. N Engl J Med 1954;250:148–9.
3. Beighton PH, Richards PR. Cardiovascular disease in air travelers. Br Heart J 1968;30:367–72.
4. Symington IS, Stack BH. Pulmonary thromboembolism after travel. Br J Dis Chest 1977;71:138–40.
5. Virchow R. Gesammelte Abhandlungen zur wissenschaftlischen. Frankfurt Meidinger 1856:227.
6. Landgraf H, Vanselow B, Schulte-Huermann D, et al. Economy class syndrome: rheology, fluid balance, and lower leg edema during a simulated 12-hour long distance flight. Aviat Space Environ Med 1994;65:930–5.
7. Moyses C, Cederholm-Williams SA, et al. Haemoconcentration and accumulation of white cells in the feet during venous stasis. Int J Microcirc Clin Exp 1987;5:311–20.
8. Egermayer P. The economy class syndrome. Problem with the assessment of risk factors for venous thromboembolism. Chest 2001;120:1407–8.
9. Geroulakos G. The risk of venous thromboembolism from air travel. The evidence is only circumstantial. Br Med J 2001;322:188.
10. Davis RM. Air travel and risk of venous thromboembolism. Pulmonary embolism after air travel may occur by chance alone. Br Med J 2001;322:1184.
11. Lapostolle F, Surget V, Borron SW, et al. Severe pulmonary embolism associated with air travel. N Engl J Med 2001;345:779–83.
12. Lapostolle F, Borron SW, Surget V, et al. Stroke associated with pulmonary embolism after air travel. Neurology 2003;60:1983–5.
13. Isayev Y, Chan RKT, Pullicino PM. "Economy class" stroke syndrome? Neurology 2002;58:960–1.
14. Foerch C, Kessler KR, Steinmetz H, Sitzer M. Economy class stroke syndrome. Neurology 2002;59:962–3.
15. Konstantinides S, Geibel A, Kasper W, et al. Patent foramen ovale is an important predictor of adverse outcome in patients with major pulmonary embolism. Circulation 1998;97:1946–51.
16. Eklof B, Kistner RL, Masuda EM, et al. Venous thromboembolism in association with prolonged air travel. Dermatol Surg 1996;22:637–41.
17. Ferrari E, Chevallier T, Chapelier A, et al. Travel as a risk factor for venous thromboembolic disease. A case control study. Chest 1999;115:440–4.
18. Belcaro G, Geroulakos G, Nicolaides AN, et al. Venous thromboembolism from air travel: the LONFLIT study. Angiology 2001;52:369–74.
19. Cesarone MR, Belcaro G, Nicolaides AN, et al. Venous thrombosis from air travel: the Lonflit 3 study. Prevention with aspirin vs low molecular heparin in high-risk subjects: a randomized trial. Angiology 2002;53:1–6.

Venous Thromboembolism from Air Travel: The LONFLIT Studies

LONFLIT1: Observation
LONFLIT2: Prevention with Stockings
LONFLIT3: Prevention with Aspirin or LMWH
LONFLIT4: Edema Evaluation
LONFLIT5: Stockings and DVT Prevention

Gianni Belcaro, Maria Rosaria Cesarone, Mark Dugall, Giulia Vinciguerra, Andrea Ledda, and Bruno M. Errichi

Introduction

There has been scientific and media interest on the risk of venous thromboembolism after long-haul flights [1]. Attention was generated recently by the death of a young girl from an episode of pulmonary embolism after a flight from Australia to the U.K. [2]. However, in 2001 there was only limited evidence for a connection between deep venous thrombosis/pulmonary embolism (DVT/PE) and flight [1] because no prospective evaluation has been performed to connect long-distance flights to thrombosis. Homans reported venous thrombosis after air travel in the 1950s (a case of a doctor who developed deep venous thrombosis) after a 14-h flight [3]. The condition was termed economy class syndrome [4]. Venous stasis, caused by prolonged sitting in a limited space, was considered to be an important causal factor. Similar circumstances such as sitting for hours in air-raid shelters in London during the Second World War had been shown to be associated with an increase in sudden death from pulmonary embolism [5]. Prolonged travel has also been reported to be associated with DVT and pulmonary embolism [6]. In a recent study including 788 patients, no increased risk of DVT among travelers was found, and only 17 had a history of previous air travel [7]. However, another study reported that a history of recent travel is found almost four times more often in patients with deep venous thrombosis than in controls [6].

Compression of veins such as the popliteal vein on the edge of the seat could be a contributing factor to venous stasis and DVT. Hemo-

Department of Biomedical Sciences, IRVINE2 Vascular Lab, Chieti University, and San Valentino Vascular Screening Project (Pe), Via Vespucci 65, 65100 Pescara, Italy

concentration, due to decreased fluid intake and water loss in the dry atmosphere of airplane cabins, has been implicated [8] together with the diuretic effect of alcohol.

Another study reported that a history of recent travel was found almost four times more often in patients with DVT than in controls [6]. In a study involving the area of Heathrow Airport in London, 61 deaths in arriving passengers over 3 years were reported and 11 were caused by pulmonary embolism. In the same period venous thromboembolism was attributable to only 1 of 28 deaths in passengers waiting to embark [9]. Biochemical changes have been reported in healthy volunteers during simulated long flights [10]. Plasma viscosity, packed cell volume, albumin concentrations, fluid balance, and lower limb size were measured. No dehydration was shown, but there was retention of an average 1150 ml fluid corresponding to an approximate 1 kg increase in body weight. This study, however, did not consider the changes in cabin-related factors such as decreased air pressure, mild hypoxia, and low humidity [11], which are difficult to reproduce in laboratory conditions. These factors clearly distinguish the effects of long-haul air travel from other types of travel. The decreased air pressure and relative hypoxia may reduce fibrinolytic activity and cause release of vein wall factors that lead venous stasis [12]. The hypobaric environment may also alter coagulation [13].

Prospective epidemiological studies are required to identify the incidence of this condition and to define subjects at higher risk. These prospective studies should screen many passengers before and after prolonged flights. Current evidence suggests that an association between asymptomatic and symptomatic DVT and long-distance flights is present and that its incidence is related to several factors.

Many airlines claim that thromboembolism usually develops after the flight when the passenger had left the airplane or that a thrombus might have been present at the beginning of the flight so that they have nothing to do with the problem. In the past no advice has been given to passengers, but based on evidence provided by recent studies and reports several airlines now give advice [14] suggesting methods to avoid stasis and circulatory problems.

Appropriate measures to prevent DVT might include general advice to passengers to stand up, and stretch, exercise, drink water, avoid putting baggage under the seat to have more leg space, and to avoid constrictive clothes. Subjects with risk factors for DVT such as a past history of DVT, hormonal treatment, malignancy, or recent surgery should carefully discuss additional protective measures with their doctors including postponing the flight. Further preventive measures might include elastic stockings or antithrombotic prophylaxis with low molecular weight heparin. At the moment there is no definitive evidence that antiplatelet agents may be effective in this condition.

This report presents findings from the LONFLIT studies, which were planned to analyze the incidence of DVT in long flights. The LONFLIT2 study prospectively evaluated the protective effects of stockings for DVT in high-risk subjects in long flights.

Part 1

Long-Haul Flights DVT (LONFLIT) Study: LONFLIT1

The aim was to evaluate the incidence of DVT in low-risk subjects after long-haul flights [15]. There were 379 low-risk subjects enrolled; 355 completed the study. Subjects had low risk for DVT with no known clinical disease and no drug treatment within 2 weeks before the flight. Their mean age was 46 years (SD 11; range, 20–80; 56% males). Patients with artificial cardiac valves, pacemakers, or chronic conditions such as diabetes, hypertension, or renal or hepatic insufficiency were excluded as well as mothers traveling with children less than 2 years of age, subjects who had undergone surgery within the previous 6 months, or those who were severely obese. Subject with a high risk for DVT including a previous episode of DVT, coagulation disorders, limitation of mobility, neoplastic disease within the previous 2 years, and large varicose veins were also excluded [16] from this group. A second group of 399 subjects classified as high risk was included; 389 completed the study (mean age, 46.4; SD 12; range, 20–80 years; 57% males). There was no difference between the two groups concerning age and sex distribution.

The definition of higher risk (according to the American College of Chest Physicians) for DVT was based on previous episode of DVT, coagulation disorders, severe obesity, or limitation of mobility due to bone or joint problems, neoplastic disease within the previous 2 years, and large varicose veins [16, 17].

The average flight duration was 12 h and 40 min (range, 10–15 h). In the history there were no other long-haul flights within the previous 2 weeks before the study flight. Subjects in flights with delay greater than 2 hours were excluded as well as those using connecting flights more than 2 h (within 10 h before the study flight). B-mode and power ultrasound were used to evaluate DVT.

Sonosite scanners with 10-MHz probes were used. Scanning was performed within 24 h after the flight. We used a questionnaire in association with the ultrasound test. Both limbs were studied. The femoral and popliteal veins were examined with compression ultrasound [16, 17].

Results

Low-risk group: Table 1 shows that were no DVTs detected in the low-risk group.

TABLE 1. LONFLIT Study 1: Evaluation of the incidence of deep venous thrombosis (DVT) in normal subjects after long-haul flights

Subjects	Number scanned	Incidence of DVT
Low risk	355	0
Limbs	710	0
High risk	389	11 (2.7%) subjects
Limbs	778	13 (1.6%) limbs
Proximal DVT		4 (1.02%) subjects (0.51%) limbs
Distal deep venous system		7 (0.77%) limbs
Superficial system		6 (0.77%) limbs

High-risk group: 11 patients (2.7%) had 13 DVT; in 2 subjects there was a femoral DVT at one side and a popliteal DVT at the opposite side. Thus, there were 13 DVTs in 778 limbs (1.6%). Four DVTs were proximal (femoral vein).

There were, in total, 19 thrombotic events (13 DVTs and 6 superficial thromboses); in total there was a thrombotic event in 4.8% of subjects and in 2.4% of limbs. Finally, 18 of 19 thromboses (94.7%) were observed in subjects sitting in window or central seats.

LONFLIT Study 2: Prospective, Randomized Evaluation of the Effect of Elastic Compression to Prevent Flight DVT

The aim was to evaluate of the incidence of DVT in high-risk subjects randomized into an elastic compression and a control group. The 833 (90.2% of 922 included) subjects who completed the study were selected according to the same flight criteria used in the previous study. Drop-outs were due to nonmedical reasons. Subjects were at high risk for venous thrombosis (the definition of high risk was equivalent to the Lonflit1 study). Mean age was 44.8 years (range, 20–80; SD 9; 57% males); there were no significant differences between control and compression groups. The average flight duration was 12h and 53min (range, 10–15h); flights were within October and December.

The ultrasound test was similar to the previous study. Scanning was made before flights (within 48h before) and within 24h after. Commercially available, below-knee, graduated compression stockings with maximum compression at the ankle of 25mmHg were used. Stockings were put on between 6 and 10h before the study flight.

The following instructions were given:

A. To move often (3min every hour)
B. To drink water (at least one glass every 2h)

TABLE 2. Results of the stockings randomization study

Randomization	DVT incidence
Controls	
422 control subjects (no stockings)	19 (4.5%) subjects
844 limbs	22 (2.6%) limbs*
	(3 in both limbs)
	(+8 superficial)
Total of thrombotic events	22 + 8 = 31 (3.6%) limbs
Stockings	
411 subjects with stockings	1 (0.24%) subjects
822 limbs	1 (0.12%) limbs*

* Difference: $P < 0.02$

C. To stretch the limbs every hour for 2 min
D. To not keep baggage in the space under the seat
E. To avoid salty snacks
F. To wear comfortable clothes

Results

In the 422 subjects in the control group we detected 22 DVTs in 19 subjects (4.5%); in 3 subjects DVT was present in both limbs. There were 8 superficial thromboses. The incidence of DVT was 4.5% considering subjects and 2.6% considering limbs. Among the 411 subjects with stockings DVT incidence was significantly decreased. There was only 1 DVT (0.24% of subjects, 0.12% of limbs; $P > 0.02$). In both groups DVTs were observed in subjects sitting in window or central (non-aisle) seats.

Comment: stockings prophylaxis decrease by 18.75 times the incidence of DVT in long-haul flights in high-risk subjects.

Combined Data from the Two Studies

In the first study, 778 subjects were included, 34 were lost to follow-up and 774 completed the protocol. In the second study, 885 were included, 52 lost, and 833 completed the protocol (411 in the stockings group).

A total of 1663 subjects were included: 1577 completed the protocol and 76 were lost and did not complete the study (they did not come to the postflight evaluation for several, nonmedical reasons; 57 for short connection time). In total, 72% of thrombotic events, including superficial thromboses, were observed in subjects sitting in window or central seats. The incidence of DVT in low-risk subjects (1.6% of limbs) appears to be very limited. The incidence of DVT is significantly reduced by wearing stockings. It is possible that instructions contributed to the lower incidence in the second study in both groups.

Part 3: LONFLIT Study 3

In this part of the study 300 subjects at high-risk for DVT were randomized into three groups to evaluate two types of prophylaxis in long-haul flights:

1. Control group: no prophylaxis.
2. Aspirin treatment group: subjects were treated with 400 mg (tablets of oral soluble aspirin; 1 dose daily for 3 days, starting 12 h before the beginning or the flight).
3. Low molecular weight heparin (LMWH) group: enoxaparine (Clexane, Rhone-Poulenc-Rorer, AVENTIS), one single dose was injected between 2 and 4 h before the flight [dose was weight adjusted, 1000 IU (equivalent to 0.1 ml) per 10 kg body weight; i.e., for a 60-kg subject a dose of 6000 units was used, and for a 80-kg person a dose of 8000 units was used].

High-risk criteria for DVT are those previously indicated in LONFLIT studies 1 and 2 as well as the scanning protocol (before–after), exclusion criteria, and suggestions to passengers (as indicated in the Lonflit2). Subjects with potential problems due to prophylaxis with aspirin or LMWH or at risk of drug interactions were excluded.

Results

Of the 100 included subjects in each group a total of 249 subjects completed the study (drop-outs due to low compliance or traveling/connections problems were 17%). Age and sex distribution were comparable in the three groups as well as risk distributions. Mean age was 47 years (range, 28–75; SD 11; 65% males).

Control group: of 82 subjects, there were 4.8% of subjects with DVT (equivalent to 3.6% of limbs) with two superficial thromboses. In total, 4.8% of limbs suffered for a thrombotic event.

Aspirin group: of 84 subjects, there were 3.6% of patients with DVT (1.8% of limbs) and two superficial thrombosis. In total, 2.9% of limbs had a thrombotic event.

LMWH group: among 82 subjects, there were no cases of DVT. One superficial thrombosis was documented. In total, only 0.61% of limbs had a thrombotic event ($P < 0.002$ in comparison with the other two groups).

In this study, 85% of DVTs were in passengers in non-aisle seats. Mild side effects were observed (gastrointestinal symptoms, which disappeared when treatment was discontinued) in 13% of patients under aspirin. No side effects were observed with LMWH.

Conclusions

Media reports have increased attention on a preventable disease [18]. British Airways now specifically mentions in their magazine that exercise prevents circulatory problems and help blood from becoming sluggish, which can happen if you sit [19]. Also, detailed verbal advice is given during the flights.

TABLE 3. Results of the low molecular weight heparin (LMWH) or aspirin randomization study: 167 high-risk subjects

Randomization	DVT incidence
Controls	
83 control subjects (no LMWH)	4 (4.82%) subjects
166 limbs	6 (3.6%) limbs*
	(2 in both limbs)
	(+2 superficial)
Total of thrombotic events	6 + 2 = 8 (4.82%) limbs
Note: Two superficial DVTs in different patients; in total 6 patients and 8 limbs were affected	
Aspirin	
84 control subjects (no LMWH)	3 (3.57%) subjects
168 limbs	3 (1.8%) limbs*
	all momolateral
	(+2 superficial)
Total of thrombotic events	3 + 2 =5
	(2.98%) limbs
Note: Two superficial thromboses in different patients; in total 5 patients and 5 limbs affected	
LMWH	
82 subjects	0 (0%) subjects
164 limbs	1 (0.12%) limbs*
	(1 superficial)
Note: One superficial thrombosis in 164 (0.61%) limbs	

* Difference: $P < 0.02$

Airlines are now under more pressure to provide medical care in flights and medical emergencies in planes [20] are more and more frequent. However, the percentages of recorded medical episodes in flight are as follow: fainting 22%, cardiac 12%, gastrointestinal 12%, seizure/stroke 11%, respiratory 11%. DVT or pulmonary embolism usually occur, if detected, in the hours after the flight. It is possible that most episodes are completely neglected by the subjects, who consider some form of swelling almost normal after sitting for so long. Further studies are required to better evaluate the incidence of DVT, cost/benefit ratio of prevention, and the efficacy of measures such as educational programs. The evaluation of pulmonary embolism requires the evaluation of larger numbers of subjects and more prolonged observations.

In LONFLIT3, aspirin prophylaxis caused a decrease in DVT incidence that was not significant, whereas one single dose of LMWH almost abolished thrombotic events. Further data are needed, but considering these observations the use of one single dose of LMWH is an important option to consider in high-risk subjects in long-haul flights if there are no contraindications.

DVT in long-haul flights is now an important safety issue [19–21] that may be addressed by several parties: travelers, travel agents, air companies, insurance companies, airport authorities, health authorities, and general practitioners. The WHO has organized a meeting to discuss the problem and potential strategies of evaluating DVT in a larger passengers sample and the effects of prophylaxis [22]. The incidence of DVT, particularly in high-risk subjects, may be high and therefore prophylaxis is advisable. On the basis of available data, elastic stockings are easy to use and the less problematic solution for prophylaxis. In high-risk subjects, one single dose of LMWH (enoxaparin) is effective in dramatically decreasing DVT risks. Exercise during flights, diet suggestion, less baggage on board to keep free leg space, and larger empty spaces on planes may help as well as suggestions from physicians not to travel (or travel differently) in conditions of particularly high risk. Patients with previous history of thrombosis are at particularly high risk to develop new episodes (as 56% of patients with a documented DVT in this study had a possible, previous episode of thrombosis in the past).

Part 2

LONFLIT4: Prevention with Stockings Prevention of Venous Thrombosis in Long-Haul Flights with Elastic Stockings: The LONFLIT 5 JAP Study

The aim of this study was to evaluate deep venous thrombosis (DVT) prophylaxis with specific elastic stockings in long-haul flights (11–13h) in high risk subjects. A group of 300 subjects was included; 76 were excluded for several problems including concomitant treatments; 224 were randomized into two groups (stockings versus controls) to evaluate prophylaxis with below-knee stockings. An exercise program was used in both groups. Scholl (UK) Flight Socks (14–17mmHg pressure at the ankle) were used. DVT was diagnosed with ultrasound scanning. The femoral, popliteal, and tibial veins were scanned before and within 90min after the flights. Of the included subjects, 102 controls and 103 treated subjects (205) completed the study. Drop-outs were due to flight connection problems.

Results

Age, sex, and risk distributions were comparable in the two groups.

In the stockings group, of 103 subjects (mean age, 42 years; SD 9; M:F = 55:48), 1 limited, distal DVT was observed (0.97%).

TABLE 4. JAP study: results table

Controls		Treatment total		*P* Value
Included subjects	114	110	224	
Completing this study	102	103	205	ns
Lost	12	7	19	
DVT	6	1	7	<0.025
%	5.8	0.97	3.12	<0.021
ITT (failures)	18/114	8/110	26/22	<0.05
%				<0.05

Intention to treat analysis detects 18 failures in the control group (12 lost to follow up + 6 thromboses) of 114 subjects (15.8%) versus 8 failures (7.3%) in the treatment group ($P < 0.05$)

In the control group (102 subjects; mean age 42.1 years; SD 10.3; M:F = 56:46), 6 subjects (5.8%) had a DVT. There were no superficial thromboses.

The difference in DVT incidence is significant ($P < 0.0025$; 6 times greater in the control group). Intention to treat analysis counts 18 failures in the control group (12 lost to follow-up +6 thromboses) of 112 subjects (15.8%) versus 8 failures (7.3%) in the treatment group ($P < 0.05$). The tolerability of the stockings was very good and there were no complaints or side effects. All events were asymptomatic.

Conclusions

Considering these observations, Scholl Flight Socks are effective in reducing the incidence of DVT in high-risk subjects.

Part 3 The Short-Haul Flights Study. The SHAPSS Study. Clots Even When You Fly Short Haul?

Preliminary Results

The epidemiological SHAPS-study (Table 5, Fig. 1) was planned with the aim of evaluating the incidence of thrombotic events (deep venous thrombosis or DVT and superficial thrombosis or SVT) in subjects traveling for less than 3 to 4 h. Another study starting in this period is the MEDFLIT study, looking at DVT during 4- to 5-h flights. The LONFLIT studies have considered longer flights, evaluating both the incidence of thrombotic events and the effects of prophylaxis on edema and swelling.

Epidemiology: in this new epidemiological study, so far, 640 subjects have been included (568 have been fully evaluated, before and after flights, completing the study). Of these subjects 179 were at medium or moderate risk for

TABLE 5. The Short-Haul (SHAPSS) study: preliminary results

Thrombotic risk level	Low	Medium	High	Total
Included	221	209	210	640
Completing the study:				
Number	188	179	201	568
Females	104	98		101
Age mean + SD	45.3 (11)	51(9)		50(8)
Age range	30–65	33–65	35–64	
Flight time (h)	3.03	2.58		2.59
DVT				
Total	*n*	0	3	9
	%	0	1.6	4.47
Proximal	*n*	0	1	2
	%	0	0.6	0.99
SVT				
	n	1	2	4
	%	0.53	1.11	1.89
Pu Emb				
	n	0	0	2
	%	0	0	0.99
Total events:				
DVT + SVT	1	5		13
	0.53	2.73		6.4
D-Dimer	ns	ns		ns (12/13)**

DVT, deep venous thrombosis; SVT, superficial vein thrombosis; Pu Emb, pulmonary embolism

** Positive (value higher than normal levels) only in 1 of 13 cases of thrombotic events

DVT (according to the risk definition of the American College of Chest Physicians) and 211 could be considered at high risk.

The incidence of DVT was 1.6% in medium risk (3 cases of 179 subjects). There were 9 DVTs of 210 high risk subjects (4.26%). In this group of subjects we also recorded two episodes of possible pulmonary embolization (PE) with positive ventilatory-perfusional scintigraphy scans (the original DVT was possibly related to the flights or aggravated by the flights).

Interventional prophylaxis: in the second part of the SHAPS study, a group at moderate to high risk were protected againts the development of DVT using specific below-knee stockings. In this part of the study 442 subjects were included: 401 completed the study (there were 41 drop-outs for several non-medical problems). In the group of controls (197 completing, 22 lost to follow-up) there were 8 DVT (1 proximal and 7 distal, below-knee thromboses). Also, 3 superficial thomboses were detected. The total incidence of thrombotic events was 5.58%.

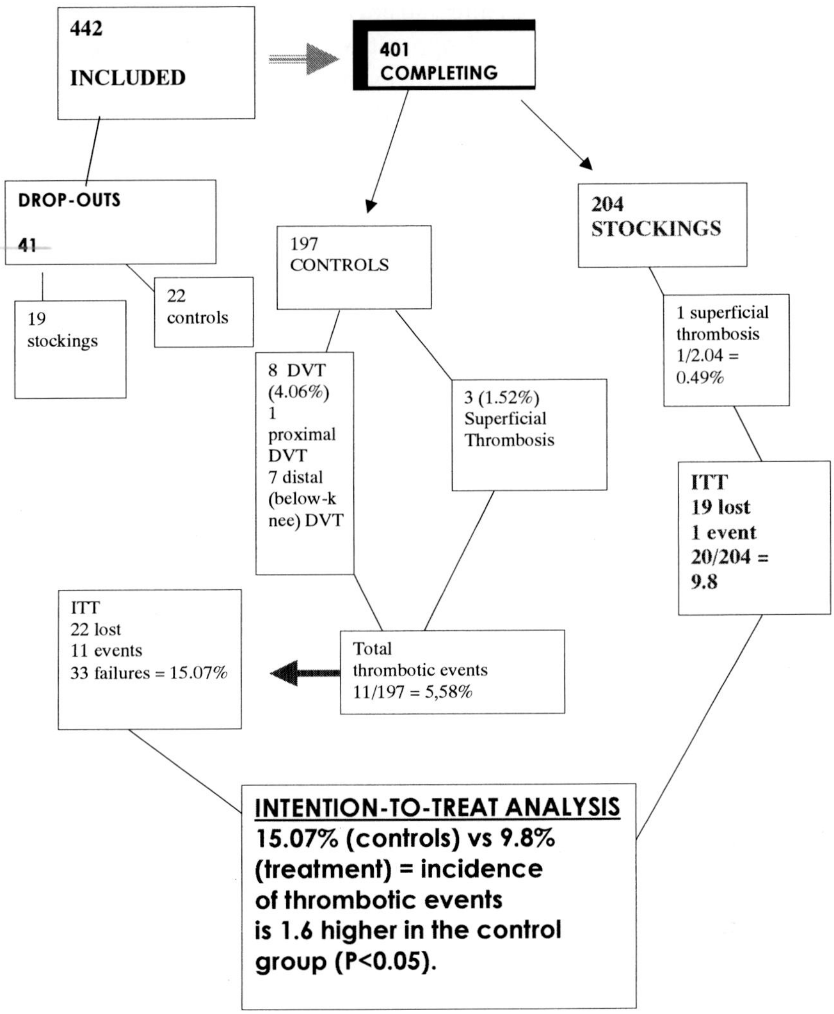

FIG. 1. Short-haul study

In the stockings group (204 subjects using below-knee stockings; 19 lost to follow-up), there was only 1 superficial thrombosis. Therefore, total incidence of thrombotic events was 0.49%.

Independent studies: these studies are organized by a group of researchers using only institutional grants and with external support from several commercial sponsors, not directly involved in the planning of the study protocol and in data analysis.

Contrast/opposition from airlines, airport authorities, and insurance companies. As it is easy to understand, opposition to this sort of studies is strong in several fields and several ways. For example, insurance companies have been requested to give compensation of the basis of evidence from our data. Airlines, particularly low-cost airllines, have contrasted in several ways the study and challenged the data. We have suggested they could redo the studies at their expense.

Studies are difficult to organize. These studies are difficult to plan and execute. Practical simple scannning with ultrasound can be made in less than 3 to 5 min for each subject using portable scanners. Subjects under evaluation do not like to wait too much in airports for scans. Three expert operators (three portable scanners) may scan some 60 to 70 subjects in 1 h. Only the most important veins (femoral, popliteal, calf veins) are imaged. Screening with more complex procedures or methods or using blood tests is more expensive, time consuming, not very practical, and may offer information only for a limited and very selected group of subjects.

Therefore, screening (i.e., for thrombophilia) is not, generally, cost effective. However, there is a major interest in planning and producing very expensive studies as this may bring very large grants. Also, there is interest dismissing previous work or in finding previous studies whether inconclusive or not-conclusive so that everything can be started over from the beginning having new grants available.

Results: for the doctors or for the public? The diffusion of these results to the general public, to increase the level of attention and interest, is very important. Any study like this, if sent to an international journal or presented at an international meeting, will require months before reaching the general public. The aim of prepublication release is to present data in an informal way widely available for discussion, comment, and analysis. Formal publication will follow in months. The prepublication material is available at www.venousforum-europe.org.

The danger: we are approaching a complex, potentially very costly problem with costly solutions, and many vendors or travel agents packing people in planes for a limited profit may be very reluctant to accept our results and suggestions or to invest in safety.

The Project "Home & Dry and No Clots": Our project H&DNC is going on with significant support from several sponsors. However, we keep full control of the planning and analysis, and our main duty in revealing data is mainly to the public and to people potentially affected by a potentially, almost fully preventable problem.

Conclusions

Some 21,000,000 passengers or even more may travel in Europe around Christmas. Some 30,000,000 per year travel on short-haul, low-cost airlines. Some 20% to 35% may be at moderate to high risk of DVT. This leads us to a number of some 200,000 to 350,000 DVTs, possibly with some pulmonary embolism. The average cost of a small, 'limited' DVT could be some 10,000 Euros per case (but it may go, considering consequences and complications, up to 100,000 for a single case). Therefore, the cost of the possible damage caused by flight-related DVTs could be as high as 1,250,000,000 Euros. The use of information, mobilization, better seating, and active prophylaxis with stockings may prevent, possibly, some 85% to 95% of these DVTs. The use of stockings, and the suggestion to avoid very cheap airlines or uncomfortable situations including long waits, sitting in airports, may achieve a significant reduction in the incidence of DVT.

Finally, we are creating an international archive of data concerning flight-related cardiovascular problems. The archive, in London, will also be available on line to the public and to researchers interested in the problem.

References

1. Geroulakos G, Hossain J, Tran T. Economy-class syndrome presenting as phlegmasia caerulea dolens. Eur J Vasc Endovasc Surg 2000;20:102–4.
2. Perry K. Blood clot kills woman after flight. Guardian 2001;23 Oct.
3. Homans J. Thrombosis of the deep leg veins due to prolonged sitting. N Engl J Med 1954;250:148–9.
4. Symington IS, Stack BHR. Pulmonary thromboembolism after travel. Br J Chest 1977;17:138–40.
5. Simpson K. Shelter deaths from pulmonary embolism. Lancet 1940;11:744.
6. Ferrari E, Chevallier T, Chapelier A, et al. Travel as a risk factor for venous thromboembolic disease: a case control study. Chest 1999;115:440–4.
7. Kraaijenhagen R, Haverkamp D, Koopman MMW, et al. Travel and risk of venous thrombosis. Lancet 2000;356:1492–3.
8. Cruickshank JM, Gorlin R, Jennett B. Air travel and thrombotic episodes: the economy class syndrome. Lancet 1988;2:497–8.
9. Sarvesvaran R. Sudden natural deaths associated with commercial air travel. Med Sci Law 1986;26:35–8.
10. Landgraf H, Vanselow B, Schulte-Huerman D, et al. Economy class syndrome: rheology fluid balance and lower leg oedema during a simulated 12-hour long-distance flight. Aviat Space Environ Med 1994;65:930–5.
11. AMA Commission on Emergency Services. Medical aspects of transportation aboard commercial aircraft. JAMA 1982;247:1007–11.
12. Gertler JP, Perry L, L'Italien G, et al. Ambient oxygen tension modulates endothelial fibrinolysis. J Vasc Surg 1993;18:939–46.
13. Bendz B, Rostrup M, Sevre K, et al. Association between acute hypobaric hypoxia and activation of coagulation in human beings. Lancet 2000;356:1657–8.

14. Webster B. Airlines tell passengers to stretch legs. Times 2001;12 Jan.
15. Geroulakos G. The risk of venous thromboembolism from air travel: the evidence is only circumstantial. Editorial. BMJ 2001;322:188.
16. Belcaro G, Stansby G, Nicolaides AN. The venous clinic. London: Imperial College Press; 1999.
17. Belcaro G, Nicolaides AN. Noninvasive investigations in vascular disease. London: Imperial College Press; 2000.
18. Calder S. Exercise your constitutional rights in the air. The Independent, 13 Jan 2001.
19. The fit flyer. High Life Magazine Dec 2000.
20. Data from USA Today Research, 2000.
21. James J. Perils of passage. Time 2001;54–59.
22. Eklof B. Report from the WHO meeting in Geneva, March 2001 (unpublished).
23. Belcaro G, Geroulakos G, Nicolaides AN, et al. Venous thromboembolism from air travel. The LONFLIT Study. Angiology 2001.

4. Prevention of Venous Thromboembolism

Incidence and the Prevention of Venous Thromboembolism in Japan: General Surgery

Masato Sakon*, Masataka Ikeda, Yasushi Hata, Rei Suzuki, Mitsugu Sekimoto, and Morito Monden

Introduction

Following the publication by Gore et al. [1] on pulmonary embolism (PE) after general surgery, the incidence of PE in Japan was thought to be low compared to that in the West. Presently, however, reports of autopsy cases lead us to believe that the incidence in Japan has increased considerably [2]. PE is one of the major causes of postoperative sudden death, and its prevention is a matter of great urgency from the standpoint of medical litigation as well, which is a growing trend. PE is usually caused by deep venous thrombosis (DVT) of the lower extremities. We could therefore say that PE prophylaxis requires DVT prophylaxis. The basic principle of prophylaxis of venous thromboembolism (VTE) is that it must be proportional to the risk, considering side effects such as hemorrhage. For that purpose, clinical data of a high level are indispensable, but in Japan there are no data that could be used as evidence. In this difficult environment, the editorial committee of the Japanese guideline for prevention of venous thromboembolism is drafting Pulmonary Embolism Guidelines for the clinical situation in Japan. The following is an introduction to the literature on postoperative PE in general surgery in Japan and a discussion of the basic concepts of the Japanese Guidelines presently in preparation.

Department of Surgery and Clinical Oncology, Graduate School of Medicine, Osaka University, E2, 2-2 Yamadaoka, Suita, Osaka 565-0871, Japan
*Present address: Department of Surgery, Nishinomiya Municipal Hospital, 8-24 Hayashida-cho, Nishinomiya, Hyogo 663-8014, Japan

Method of Searching for Publications

Using the key words "surgery" and "pulmonary embolism" or "thromboembolism," we searched for relevant papers in PubMed and Japana Centra Revuo Medicina (Tokyo) editions from 1985 to 2002. We chose 26 publications and their reference materials and divided the data into abdominal, thoracic, or general (abdominal/thoracic) surgery for review.

Incidence of Postoperative PE in General Surgery

The incidence of symptomatic PE (clinical PE) in Japanese surgical patients is summarized in Table 1. Clinical PE has a total incidence of 0.33% (116/35,369). There is considerable variability among the different papers, ranging from 0.08% to 2.3%. Thoracic surgery shows a higher trend at 1.2% compared to abdominal surgery (0.32%). There were, however, no reports concerning cardiovascular surgery. Analysis of the 26 publications that our search yielded showed that studies with a larger number of cases tended to have a lower incidence of PE and studies with fewer cases tended to have a higher incidence. Because PE diagnosis is difficult, it is possible that some PE patients in the larger studies may have been overlooked and never diagnosed. When classified according to the 6th American College of Chest Physicians (6th ACCP) consensus recommendations [3], abdominal surgery had a low, and thoracic surgery a moderate, risk level. The overall mortality rate of PE was 0.08% (26/31,734), 0.34% in thoracic surgery and 0.03% in abdominal surgery, again showing a higher incidence in the former. These data reveal, however, that once PE occurs the mortality rate is very high (31%, 26/85 cases), demonstrating the importance of prevention (Table 2). If we apply the 6th ACCP consensus recommendations to the incidence of fatal PE in Japan, thoracic surgery showed a moderate, and abdominal surgery a low, risk level, similar to the results with clinical PE.

TABLE 1. The incidence of clinical pulmonary embolism (PE) in the Japanese surgical population

	No. of patients	No. of PE patients	Incidence (%)
Thoracic surgery	3,825	44	1.15
Abdominal surgery	11,890	36	0.32
Abdominal and thoracic surgery	19,654	36	0.18
Total	35,369	116	0.33

TABLE 2. The incidence of fatal pulmonary embolism (PE) in the Japanese surgical population

	No. of patients	No. of death (no. of PE patients)	Mortality rate in PE patients (%)	Incidence of fatal PE (%)
Thoracic surgery	2,975	10 (27)	37.0	0.34
Abdominal surgery	9,105	3 (22)	13.6	0.03
Thoracic and abdominal surgery	19,654	13 (36)	36.1	0.07
total	31,734	26 (85)	30.6	0.08

Incidence in Patients Undergoing Cancer Surgery

The number of studies that strictly distinguished PE in cancer and noncancer surgery was small, with only five studies reported [4–8]. The overall incidence of PE in cancer surgery was 1.6% (Table 3). In Japanese cancer patients undergoing surgery, the incidence of PE was about eight times higher than in nonmalignant surgical patients (0.2%). In cancer patients, more extensive surgery is generally performed and the operation times are often longer compared with surgery for benign diseases. In addition, cancer tissues produce procoagulants [9, 10]. These underlying mechanisms may contribute to the development of VTE in cancer surgery. Most of the reported incidences in cancer surgery corresponded to a moderate to high level of risk as defined in the 6th ACCP consensus recommendations. Most of these cancer patients undergoing surgery have the three major risk factors (cancer, age older than 40 years, major surgery) and would be classified at the highest level of risk in the ACCP consensus recommendations. Therefore, the risk of the Japanese surgical population may be one or two levels lower than that of Western surgical populations.

TABLE 3. The incidence of pulmonary embolism (PE) in Japanese patients undergoing cancer surgery

Cancer	No. of patients	No. of PE patients	Incidence (%)	Risk level classified according to 6th ACCP guideline
Lung [4]	102	3	2.94	High
Esophagus [5]	745	24	3.22	High
Stomach [6, 7]	1176	13	1.11	Moderate
Pancreas [7]	78	3	3.85	High
Colon [7, 8]	1059	6	0.57	Low
Rectum [7]	193	3	1.55	Moderate
Total	3353	52	1.55	Moderate
Noncancer [6, 7]	2014	4	0.20	Low

ACCP, American College of Chest Physicians

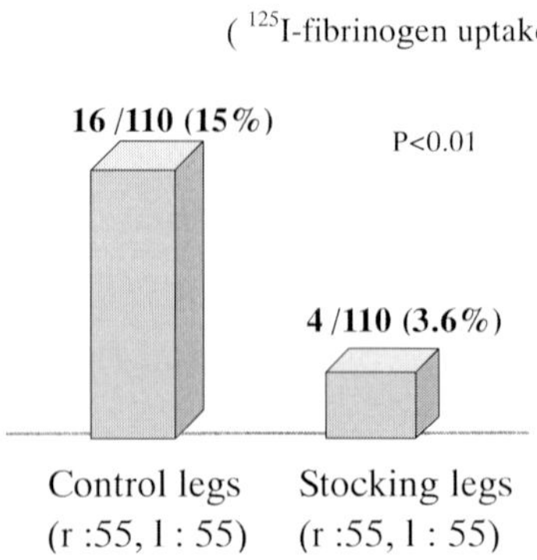

Fig. 1. Effect of gradient compression stockings on deep-vein thrombosis (DVT) in general surgery [11]

TABLE 4. Effect of mechanical prophylaxis for pulmonary embolism (PE) in Japanese surgical population

	Without prophylaxis (%) (PE cases/total cases)	With prophylaxis (%) (PE cases/total cases)	*P* value
IPC	0.60 (16/2,670)	0.10 (1/964)	0.055
ES + IPC	0.18 (26/14,732)	0.04 (3/8036)	0.17

IPC, intermittent pneumatic compression; ES, elastic stockings

Studies on Thromboprophylaxis in Japanese Surgical Patients

There are no reports in Japan on thromboprophylaxis using anticoagulants such as heparin and warfarin. There are, however, a few papers on the use of mechanical prophylactic methods such as elastic stockings (ES) and intermittent pneumatic compression (IPC). Inada et al. [11] conducted ^{125}I-fibrinogen uptake tests and reported that the incidence of DVT decreased from 15% to 3.6% with the use of ES (Fig. 1). However, this would not be sufficient prophylaxis in high-risk patients. With regard to IPC, there are eight reports, with or without the combined use of ES, and only one showed statistically significant results. On the whole, however, regardless of whether ES was used, IPC could reduce the incidence of clinical PE to 1/4 to 1/6 (Table 4).

Basic Concept in Japanese Guidelines for Venous Thromboembolism in General Surgery

PE is a common occurrence in general surgery and has an extremely high mortality rate once it occurs. Furthermore, litigation cases involving the onset of PE have recently increased in Japan. Because the incidence of PE in Japan differs from that of the West, Western prophylaxis guidelines cannot be directly applied to Japanese general surgical patients. Guidelines suitable for

TABLE 5. Sixth ACCP recommendations and Japanese guideline for venous thromboembolism (VTE) in general surgical patients

Sixth ACCP guidelines:

Risk level	PE (%)	Examples	Prophylaxis
Low	0.2	Minor surgery: <40 years or risk factor (−)	Aggressive mobilization
Moderate	1–2	Minor surgery: risk factor (+) Nonmajor surgery: 40–60 years + risk factor (−) Major surgery: <40 years + risk factor (−)	ES, IPC, LMWH, or LDUH (q12h)
High	2–4	Nonmajor surgery: >60 years or risk factor (+) Major surgery: >40 years or risk factor (+)	IPC, LMWH, or LDUH (q8h)
Highest	4–10	Major surgery: >40 years + (prior VTE, cancer, or hypercoagulable state)	LMWH, warfarin, IPC/ES+LDUH/LMWH, or ADH

Japanese guideline:

Risk level	PE (%)	Examples	Prophylaxis
Low	0.2	Nonmajor surgery: <60 years Major surgery: <40 years	Aggressive mobilization
Moderate	1–2	Nonmajor surgery: >60 years or risk factor (+) Major surgery: >40 years or risk factor (+)	ES, IPC
High	2–4	Major surgery: >40 years + cancer	IPC or LDUH (q8–12h)
Highest	4–10	Major surgery: prior VTE or thrombophilia	LDUH + IPC, or LDUH + ES[a]

LMWH, low molecular weight heparin; LDUH, low-dose unfractionated heparin; ADH, adjusted-dose heparin

[a] ADH or oral anticoagulant can be chosen, if necessary

Japan are therefore of vital importance. However, Japan is totally lacking in prospective and randomized clinical data on the prevention or incidence of PE. In other words, Japan has no evidence regarding PE incidence. In this situation, to generate guidelines that are evidence-based as much as possible, we have no recourse but to effectively utilize the evidence-based 6th ACCP consensus recommendations (Table 5). In concrete terms, we will use four categories from low risk to highest risk, based on the 6th ACCP consensus recommendations, and apply the prophylaxis recommended for each risk level to Japanese patients according to their PE occurrence status. By this methodology we not only can avail ourselves of the wealth of evidence regarding prevention in the ACCP guidelines, but also carry out risk evaluation using the same categories as the West. Namely, we will be able to have risk and prophylaxis data compatible with those of the West. Although the existing Japanese data are limited, as already mentioned, the PE incidence of Japanese general surgical patients corresponds more or less to one lower rank in the 6th ACCP guidelines (see Table 3). Therefore, the prophylaxis guidelines for Japanese general surgical patients are adjusted one rank lower than the 6th ACCP guidelines (see Table 5).

Conclusions

The incidence of PE in Japanese general surgical patients is not low, and the mortality rate is high once PE occurs. In such a situation the establishment of methods of prevention based on greater evidence is urgently required. Because of the lack of sufficient evidence, however, we have no recourse but to recommend the 6th ACCP guidelines in accordance with the incidence in Japan. Data collection in line with these guidelines and revision of the guidelines based on the data are important tasks for the future.

References

1. Gore I, Hirst AE, Tanaka K. Myocardial infarction and thromboembolism. Arch Intern Med 1964;113:323–30.
2. Ito M. Pathology of pulmonary embolism (in Japanese with English abstract). Kokyu to Jyunkan (Respiration and Circulation) 1991;39:567–72.
3. Geerts WH, Heit JA, Clagett GP, et al. Prevention of venous thromboembolism. Chest 2001;119:132S–75S.
4. Naruke Y, Oizumi H, Fujishima T, Shiono S, Shimazaki Y. Hypoxia after lung cancer surgery: the possibility of pulmonary embolism (abstract in Japanese). Haigan (Jpn J Lung Cancer) 2000;40:446.
5. Tsutsumi K, Udagawa H, Kajiyama Y, et al. Pulmonary thromboembolism after surgery for esophageal cancer: its features and prophylaxis. Surg Today 2001;30:416–20.
6. Tsutsumi K, Tsurumaru M, Udagawa H, et al. Studies on pulmonary embolism after surgery for esophageal cancer (in Japanese). Nihon Gekakeirengo Gakkaishi (J Jpn Coll Surg) 1994;19:82–6.
7. Sakon M. Perioperative prophylaxis of pulmonary embolism in general surgery (in Japanese). Heart View 2002;6:117–21.
8. Ishida H, Tatsuta M, Masutani S, et al. Postoperative complications and mortality following elective surgery for colorectal cancer (in Japanese). Nihon Gekakeirengo Gakkaishi (J Jpn Coll Surg) 2002;27:233–7.
9. Kwaan HC, Parmar S, Wang J. Pathogenesis of increased risk of thrombosis in cancer. Semin Thromb Hemost 2003;29:283–90.
10. Sutherland DE, Weitz IC, Liebman HA. Thromboembolic complications of cancer: epidemiology, pathogenesis, diagnosis, and treatment. Am J Hematol 2003;72:43–52.
11. Inada K, Shirai N, Hayashi M, et al. Postoperative deep venous thrombosis in Japan: incidence and prophylaxis. Am J Surg 1983;145:775–9.

Incidence and Prevention of Venous Thromboembolism in Orthopedic Surgery in Japan

Satoru Fujita

Introduction

The rate of venous thromboembolism (VTE) in orthopedic surgery is higher in the lower extremities than in other areas because of the long rest period after surgery and impaired blood flow in the legs. According to the 6th ACCP Guidelines [1], the rate of occurrence of postoperative VTE is very high in the West. The incidence of deep venous thromboembolism (DVT) is 45%–57% in total hip replacement (THR), 40%–84% in total knee replacement (TKR), and 36%–60% in hip fracture surgery. The incidence of postoperative pulmonary thromboembolism (PTE) is reported to be as follows: THR, 0.7%–30%; TKR, 1.8%–7%; and hip fracture surgery, 4.3%–24%. The Guidelines therefore recommend preventive anticoagulant therapy using low molecular weight heparin or warfarin in these kinds of orthopedic surgeries.

In Japan, there are few epidemiological surveys of the incidence of VTE after orthopedic surgery, and at present we have no guidelines for VTE prevention. Therefore, the method of prevention is decided by the individual institution or clinician. Two methods that are generally used in Japan after major orthopedic surgery such as THR or TKR are elastic stockings and intermittent pneumatic compression (IPC). Prophylactic anticoagulant therapy is not as prevalent as in the West, but low-dose unfractionated heparin is frequently considered when the patient to receive surgery is obese or has thrombotic risk factors. However, in Japan low-dose unfractionated heparin is usually administered at a dose of 2500 units given subcutaneously twice a day, which is lower than the Western dosage of 5000 units two to three times a day.

Department of Orthopaedic Surgery, Takarazuka Daiichi Hospital 19-5 Kogetsu-cho, Takarazuka, Hyogo 665-0832, Japan

TABLE 1. Demographic and operative characteristics of the patients

	THR	TKR	Cervical spine	Lumbar spine
No. of patients	71	51	54	49
Sex (M/F)	7/64	9/42	30/24	29/20
Age (average, years)	63	70	62	57
BMI (average, years)	23.5	23.7	23.1	23.5
Operative time (average, min)	103	101	144	166
Prophylaxis	ES	ES	—	—

THR, total hip replacement; TKR, total knee replacement; BMI, body mass index; ES, elastic stockings

TABLE 2. Incidence of deep venous thrombosis (DVT)

	THR (%)	TKR (%)	Cervical spine (%)	Lumbar spine (%)
Overall	32.4	60.8	5.6	26.5
Proximal DVT	8.4	9.6	0	1.0
Distal DVT	12.8	32.3	3.7	14.3

THR, total hip replacement; TKR, total knee replacement

Incidence of Venous Thromboembolism

First of all, let me introduce a Japanese study on DVT incidence [2]. The subjects were 225 patients who underwent artificial joint replacement surgery of the lower extremities or surgery of the posterior spine at Osaka Prefectural Hospital between July 1997 and October 1999. There were 71 THR, 51 TKR, 54 cervical spine, and 49 lumbar spine cases (Table 1). The method used for the study was venography of both legs 1–2 weeks after surgery to examine for DVT. Postoperative use of anticoagulants or IPC was prohibited.

Survey Data

The incidence of DVT was THR, 32.4%; TKR, 60.8%; cervical spine, 5.6%; and lumbar spine, 26.5%, demonstrating that with the exception of cervical spine surgery, the incidence of postoperative DVT in Japan is high. In THR and TKR in particular, proximal DVT, which has a high risk of PTE, was about 10% (Table 2). A comparison of the treated and untreated extremities in artificial joint replacement surgery showed the incidence of DVT in THR to be 25.4% in the treated leg and 15.5% in the untreated leg, and in TKR the ratio was 58.8% versus 11.8%, showing a high incidence of DVT in the TKR-treated limb ($P < 0.01$). A comparison of the left and right lower extremities after spinal

TABLE 3. Incidence of venous thromboembolism (VTE) after total hip replacement

Author	Year	Total DVT	Proximal DVT	Clinical PE	Fatal PE
Shibayama [3]	1994			0.1% (1/739)	0% (0/739)
Shimagaki [4]	1996			0.2% (1/636)	0.2% (1/636)
Kitajima [5]	1999			1.4% (1/71)	0% (0/71)
Oura [6]	1999			0.8% (4/514)	0.4% (2/514)
Yanagimoto [7]	1999			2.2% (11/493)	0% (0/493)
Tamai [8]	1999	33.3% (3/9)			
Murayama [9]	2000			0.7% (1/136)	0% (0/136)
Fujita [10]	2000	22.6% (37/164)	9.8% (16/164)	0.1% (2/164)	0% (0/164)
Fujita [11]	2000	27.4% (17/62)	4.8% (3/62)	0% (0/62)	0% (0/62)
Yamauchi [12]	2000			0.8% (1/123)	0.8% (1/123)
Kobayashi [13]	2000			0.1% (1/1,061)	0% (0/1,061)
Kajitani [14]	2000	42.6% (20/47)	31.9% (15/47)		
Takano [15]	2001			1.5% (3/202)	1.0% (2/202)
Kokubo [16]	2001			2.4% (3/127)	0.8% (1/127)
Nishiyama [17]	2001			1.7% (3/176)	0% (0/176)
Total		27.3% (77/282)	12.5% (34/273)	0.7% (32/4,504)	0.2% (7/4,504)

PE, pulmonary embolism

surgery showed the following: cervical spine: left side, 5.6%; right side, 1.9%; lumbar spine: left side, 20.4%; right side, 12.2%. These results show a greater tendency toward the occurrence of DVT on the left side compared to the right side after spinal surgery. This tendency is considered to be a reflection of anatomical characteristics (the left common iliac vein is easily compressed by the right common iliac artery when they cross).

To obtain data on the incidence of postoperative VTE in the orthopedic surgery field, I reviewed all the relevant Japanese literature of the past 10 years (1993–2002). DVT was diagnosed by venography, and only symptomatic PTE cases were considered. Cases of postoperative anticoagulant therapy or IPC use were excluded.

Summary of Data

The greatest number of reports concern THR, with 4 on DVT [8, 10, 11, 14] and 13 on PTE [3–7, 9–13, 15–17]. The incidence of post-THR VTE calculated from all the reports is as follows: total DVT, 27.3%; proximal DVT, 12.5%; clinical PTE, 0.7%; and fatal PTE, 0.2% (Table 3).

There are also relatively numerous reports about TKR, with four on DVT [10, 11, 14, 18] and six on PTE [9–12, 15, 19]. The incidence of postoperative VTE calculated from all the reports is as follows: total DVT, 50.5%; proximal

Table 4. Incidence of VTE after total knee replacement

Author	Year	Total DVT	Proximal DVT	Clinical PE	Fatal PE
Kawakubo [18]	1999	80.0% (8/10)			
Murayama [9]	2000			0.9% (3/320)	0% (0/320)
Fujita [10]	2000	48.6% (67/138)	14.5% (20/138)	1.4% (2/138)	0% (0/138)
Fujita [11]	2000	50.0% (17/34)	11.8% (4/34)	0% (0/34)	0% (0/34)
Yamauchi [12]	2000			0% (0/89)	0% (0/89)
Sugita [19]	2000			0% (0/32)	0% (0/32)
Kajitani [14]	2000	50.0% (12/24)	8.3% (2/24)		
Takano [15]	2001			2.1% (3/144)	0% (0/144)
Total		50.5% (104/206)	13.3% (26/196)	1.1% (8/757)	0% (0/757)

Table 5. Incidence of VTE after surgery for hip fracture

Author	Year	Total DVT	Proximal DVT	Clinical PE	Fatal PE
Tamai [8]	1999	26.7% (4/15)			
Ishibashi [20]	2001			3.8% (1/26)	0% (0/26)
Kokubo [16]	2001			0.8% (5/615)	0% (0/615)
Abe [21]	2002			2.9% (9/307)	1.0% (3/307)
Shiota [22]	2002	50.0% (18/36)	30.6% (11/36)		
Total		43.7% (22/51)	30.6% (11/36)	1.6% (15/948)	0.3% (3/948)

DVT, 13.3%; clinical PTE, 1.1%; and fatal PTE, 0% (Table 4). The incidence of total DVT after TKR exceeded 50%, an extremely high rate.

There are few reports on the incidence of VTE after hip fracture surgery, with only two on DVT [8, 22] and three on PTE [16, 20, 21]. The incidence was as follows: total DVT, 43.7%; proximal DVT, 30.6%; clinical PTE, 1.6%; and fatal PTE, 0.3% (Table 5). Proximal DVT and clinical PTE occurred at high rates after hip fracture surgery.

In the case of surgery of the pelvis and lower extremities, there are no reports on DVT incidence and ten reports on PTE [3, 23–31], with the following results: clinical PTE, 1.3%; and fatal PTE, 0.1% (Table 6). Orthopedic surgery of the lower extremities is believed to generate about 1% of the case of PTE.

There are few reports on spinal surgery, with only one concerning DVT [33] and five on PTE [29, 30, 32–34]. The results are total DVT, 15.5%; proximal DVT, 0.9%; clinical PTE, 0.9%; and fatal PTE, 0.1% (Table 7). The incidence of DVT after spinal surgery may be low compared to surgery of the lower extremities, but the incidence of PTE, 0.9%, is comparable.

TABLE 6. Incidence of VTE after surgery of pelvis and lower extremity

Author	Year	Surgery	Clinical PE	Fatal PE
Shibayama [3]	1994	Chiari pelvic osteotomy	2.2% (14/634)	0.3% (2/634)
Hiraga [23]	1997	Pelvis and lower extremity	2.0% (2/98)	0% (0/98)
Okawa [24]	1998	Lower extremity	0.6% (3/520)	0% (0/520)
Tahara [25]	1999	Hip joint	0.3% (2/651)	0% (0/651)
Okawa [26]	1999	Chiari pelvic osteotomy	1.3% (1/80)	0% (0/80)
Hirota [27]	2000	Pelvis and lower extremity	1.2% (2/173)	0% (0/173)
Mabuchi [28]	2001	Hip joint	3.6% (2/56)	0% (0/56)
Kudo [29]	2001	Hip joint	1.2% (3/251)	
Yonekura [30]	2001	Lower extremity	1.5% (4/263)	
Abe [31]	2001	Lower extremity	1.6% (7/442)	
Total			1.3% (40/3,168)	0.1% (2/2,212)

TABLE 7. Incidence of VTE after surgery of spine

Author	Year	Total DVT	Proximal DVT	Clinical PE	Fatal PE
Nishizawa [32]	1996			0.4% (1/261)	0% (0/261)
Oda [33]	2000	15.5% (17/110)	0.9% (1/110)	0% (0/110)	0% (0/110)
Tateno [34]	2001			0.4% (3/852)	0.1% (1/852)
Yonekura [30]	2001			2.3% (9/397)	0% (0/397)
Kudo [29]	2001			1.5% (4/263)	
Total		15.5% (17/110)	0.9% (1/110)	0.9% (17/1,883)	0.1% (1/1,620)

Prevention of Venous Thromboembolism

Because data on VTE prophylaxis are limited in Japan, we need to establish levels of risk and corresponding preventive measures in accordance with the 6th ACCP Guidelines. Proximal DVT and clinical PTE are the elements used to determine risk levels.

Compiling the survey results, we find that proximal DVT after THR, TKR, and hip fracture surgery is more than 10%, representing the highest risk, but the PTE incidence in all the operations that were reevaluated was approximately 1%, corresponding to a moderate risk (Table 8). It is therefore appropriate to classify THR, TKR, and hip fracture surgery in the high risk level and surgery of the pelvis, lower extremity, and spine in the moderate-risk level.

Low molecular weight heparin cannot be used in Japan for VTE prevention. Because anticoagulant therapy is still not generally used for prophylaxis, I would recommend the use of low-dose unfractionated heparin, limited to high- and highest risk levels of surgery. Based on these considerations, the

TABLE 8. Incidence of VTE after orthopedic surgery

Surgery	Proximal DVT	Clinical PE
THR	12.5% (8.8%–17.0%)	0.7% (0.5%–1.0%)
TKR	13.3% (8.9%–18.8%)	1.1% (0.5%–2.1%)
Hip fracture	30.6% (16.3%–48.1%)	1.6% (0.9%–2.6%)
Pelvis and lower extremity	Unclear	1.3% (0.9%–1.7%)
Spine	0.9% (0%–5.0%)	0.9% (0.5%–1.4%)

Figures in parentheses are 95% confidence interval

TABLE 9. Risk level of VTE and prophylaxis

Risk level	Surgery	Prophylaxis
Low	Upper extremity	Early mobilization
Moderate	Spine	ES or IPC
	Pelvis	
	Lower extremity	
High	THR	IPC or LDUH
	TKR	
	Hip fracture	
Highest	High-risk patients with risk	(LDUH + IPC) or (LDUH + ES)

Risk factor, history of VTE and/or thrombophilia
THR, total hip replacement; TKR, total knee replacement; ES, elastic stockings; IPC, intermittent pneumatic compression; LDUH, low-dose unfractionated heparin

risk levels of VTE and the corresponding prophylaxis for orthopedic surgery in Japan are summarized in Table 9. Prophylaxis for THR, TKR, and hip fracture surgery, which are high risk, consists of IPC or low-dose unfractionated heparin. The recommended low-dose unfractionated heparin is 5000 units b.i.d. If the THR, TKR, or hip fracture surgery patients have congenital thrombotic risk factors or a history of thromboembolism, they are considered to be at the highest risk, and appropriate prophylaxis would be low-dose unfractionated heparin and IPC or low-dose unfractionated heparin and elastic stockings. Prophylaxis for moderate-risk surgery, that is, pelvis, lower extremity, or spine, would be elastic stockings or IPC. Surgery of the upper extremities does not require special preventive measures as patients are able to walk immediately after or at least the day after the operation.

Hip fracture is highly prevalent among the elderly, many of whom are unable to receive anticoagulant therapy because of various complications. Shiota et al. [22] reported that the DVT incidence was 14.3% in patients who were operated on within 48 h after injury, whereas it was 58.6% when more than 48 h had elapsed before surgery. Kato et al. [35] reported that DVT incidence was 5.3% according to ultrasound of the lower extremities in patients who were ambulatory within 6 days after injury, whereas it was 26.3% in patients who were bedridden for more than 7 days. In hip fracture patients, therefore, early surgery and early mobilization are essential for VTE prevention.

Future Prospects

Clinical trials of low molecular weight heparin (enoxaparin) and pentasaccharide (fondaparinux) have been completed in Japan. These drugs are expected to be available for prophylactic use in the near future.

Japan is finally realizing an environment in which systematic PTE prevention can be carried out. As data on prevention gradually accumulate, further progress in this field can be expected.

References

1. Geerts WH, Heit JA, Clagett GP, et al. Prevention of venous thromboembolism. Chest 2001;119:132S–5S.
2. Fujita S. Venous thromboembolism in orthopedic surgery (in Japanese). Jpn Soc Biorheol 2001;15:33–4.
3. Shibayama K, Higuchi F, Shinami N, et al. Pulmonary embolism after hip surgery (in Japanese). Rinsho Seikei Geka (Clin Orthop Surg) 1994;29:999–1006.
4. Shimagaki S, Matsubara T, Narisawa H, et al. Two cases of fatal pulmonary embolism after total hip replacement (in Japanese). Arch Niigata Soc Orthop Surg 1996;12:121–4.
5. Kitajima I, Tachibana S, Hirota Y, et al. The incidence of pulmonary embolism following total hip arthroplasty (in Japanese). Seikeigeka (Orthop Surg) 1999;50:1287–90.
6. Oura K, Shimada W, Kikuchi K, et al. Pulmonary embolism after total hip replacement (in Japanese). Jpn Soc Replacement Arthroplasty 1999;29:241–2.
7. Yanagimoto S. Pulmonary embolism after total hip arthroplasty (in Japanese). J Musculoskeletal System 1999;12:889–93.
8. Tamai K, Nakajima T, Kobayashi T, et al. Deep venous thrombosis after the operations of the hip (in Japanese). Hip Joint 1999;25:89–93.
9. Murayama T, Sunahara N, Maeda M, et al. Pulmonary embolism in total hip and knee arthroplasty patients (in Japanese). Kyusyu J Rheumatol 2000;19:136–8.
10. Fujita S, Hirota S, Oda T, et al. Deep venous thrombosis after total hip or total knee arthroplasty in patients in Japan. Clin Orthop 2000;375:168–74.
11. Fujita S, Fuji T, Mitsii T, et al. Prospective multicenter study on prevalence of deep vein thrombosis after total hip or knee arthroplasty (in Japanese). Seikeigeka (Orthop Surg) 2000;51:745–9.
12. Yamauchi K, Hasegawa K, Sakano M, et al. Incidence of symptomatic deep-vein thrombosis after hip and knee arthroplasties (in Japanese). Cent Jpn J Orthop Traumatol 2000;43:1297–8.
13. Kobayashi S, Saito N, Urayama H, et al. Prevalence of deep vein thrombosis after total hip arthroplasty (in Japanese). Cent Jpn J Orthop Traumatol 2000;43:1299–300.
14. Kajitani M, Sato T, Shiota N, et al. Deep vein thrombosis after total hip and knee arthroplasty (in Japanese). Cent Jpn J Orthop Traumatol 2000;43:1301–2.

15. Takano T, Ito K, Sano K, et al. Pulmonary embolism following artificial arthroplasty of the lower extremities (in Japanese). Kanto J Orthop Traumatol 2001;32:17–24.
16. Kokubo Y, Yamazaki T, Shiba T, et al. The clinical usefulness of inferior vena cava filter for the treatment of pulmonary thromboembolism after hip surgery (in Japanese). Kanto J Orthop Traumatol 2001;32:30–5.
17. Nishiyama T, Kakunan K, Sato T, et al. Pulmonary embolism after total hip arthroplasty (3 cases) (in Japanese). Cent Jpn J Orthop Traumatol 2001;44:687–8.
18. Kawakubo M, Sekiguchi O, Matsuzaki K, et al. Deep vein thrombosis after total knee arthroplasty: effect of preoperative low molecular weight heparin (in Japanese). J Jpn Orthop Assoc 1999;73:S501.
19. Sugita J, Hashimoto J, Kobayashi N, et al. The incidence of pulmonary embolism after total knee arthroplasty and the effect of early medical therapy (in Japanese). J Jpn Orthop Assoc 2000;74:S845.
20. Ishibashi H, Yamamoto S, Ono T, et al. Incidence of deep vein thrombosis and pulmonary embolism after operative treatment for hip fractures examined with perfusion scintigram (in Japanese). Kanto J Orthop Traumatol 2001;32:13–16.
21. Abe Y, Nakano T, Ochi R, et al. The pulmonary embolism of 307 cases of hip fractures (in Japanese). Kossetsu (J Jpn Soc Fracture Repair) 2002;24:1–4.
22. Shiota N, Sato T, Matsuo M, et al. Incidence, diagnosis and treatment of deep vein thrombosis and pulmonary embolism after the operation for the fracture of proximal femur (in Japanese). Kossetsu (J Jpn Soc Fracture Repair) 2002;24:83–7.
23. Hiraga Y, Tachibana S, Hirota Y, et al. Prospective study of pulmonary embolism after surgeries of the lower extremities (in Japanese). East Jpn J Orthop Traumatol 1997;9:399–402.
24. Okawa T, Yamauchi K, Morizane K, et al. Three cases of pulmonary thrombo-embolism in knee or ankle joint surgery (in Japanese). Seikeigeka (Orthop Surg) 1998;49:1545–8.
25. Tahara Y, Kodera M, Ishii Y. Two cases of pulmonary embolism after hip surgery (in Japanese). Hip Joint 1999;25:112–15.
26. Okawa T, Higuchi F, Akashi H, et al. Prevention of pulmonary embolism after hip surgery (in Japanese). J Musculoskeletal System 1999;12:877–82.
27. Hirota Y, Tachibana S. The incidence of pulmonary embolism following lower extremity surgery (in Japanese). J Joint Surg 2000;19:49–54.
28. Mabuchi A, Moro T, Nagai I, et al. Prevention of pulmonary embolism in hip surgery with venous foot pump and minidose warfarin (in Japanese). Kanto J Orthop Traumatol 2001;32:45–8.
29. Kudo T, Inoue Y, Sugano N, et al. Pulmonary embolism (in Japanese). Seikeigeka (Orthop Surg) 2001;52:1023–9.
30. Yonekura T, Okajima K, Suguro T. Diagnosis and risk factors for pulmonary thromboembolism following spinal surgery (in Japanese). Orthop Surg Traumatol 2001;44:1203–8.
31. Abe K, Yamamoto K, Nemoto T, et al. Three cases of pulmonary embolism following total hip arthroplasty (in Japanese). J Tokyo Med College 2001;59:159–64.
32. Nishizawa T, Fujimura Y, Takahata T, et al. Complications of anterior interbody fusion for lumbar degenerative disease (in Japanese). East Jpn J Clin Orthop 1996;8:22–5.
33. Oda T, Fuji T, Kato Y, et al. Deep venous thrombosis after spinal surgery. Spine 2000;25:2962–7.
34. Tateno K, Morishita M, Kanzaki K, et al. Clinical analysis for pulmonary thromboembolism after spine surgery (in Japanese). Kanto J Orthop Traumatol 2001;32:3–9.
35. Kato H, Matsuda M. Incidence and management of deep vein thrombosis in patients with hip fracture (in Japanese). Seikei-Geka Kango 2002;7:33–6.

Incidence of Venous Thromboembolism and Guidelines for Thromboembolism Prophylaxis in Japan: Obstetrics and Gynecology

Takao Kobayashi

Introduction

Venous thromboembolism (VTE), which had been considered a relatively rare disease in Japan, has been on the increase in recent years as eating habits have become more similar to those of the West. Patients with VTE have a clinical problem in which there is deep venous thrombosis (DVT) or pulmonary thromboembolism (PTE) caused by DVT. Pregnancy is conducive to VTE for the following reasons: (1) enhanced coagulation, reduced fibrinolysis, and platelet activation; (2) the venous smooth muscle relaxation effect of estrogen/progesterone; (3) compression of the iliac vein and inferior vena cava by the enlarged gravid uterus; and (4) vascular (particularly endothelial) disorders of the iliac vein region caused by surgical interventions such as cesarean section and retention of blood caused by postoperative immobilization.

In the field of obstetrics, the diseases and conditions that are risk factors are middle-aged pregnancy, prolonged immobilization due to severe preeclampsia, placenta previa, hyperemesis, threatened abortion or threatened premature labor, placental abruption, delivery by cesarean section, and marked varix of the lower limbs. In the field of gynecology, the risk factors are surgery for giant uterine myoma, giant ovarian tumor, ovarian cancer, uterine cancer, and severe pelvic adhesion. Other patients at risk are those with ovarian hyperstimulation syndrome (OHSS), patients taking oral contraceptives, and postmenopausal patients receiving hormone replacement therapy. Many cases that require long operations with lymphatic resection, massive bleeding, or transfusions are also at risk [1–4].

Shinshu University School of Health Sciences, 3-1-1 Asahi, Matsumoto, Nagano 390-8621, Japan

In this chapter, I have reviewed the incidence of thrombosis in obstetrics and gynecology in Japan and have established guidelines for the prevention of venous thromboembolism.

Methods

1. A survey of the incidence of obstetric and gynecological thrombosis in Japan, focusing on university and general hospitals. This is an ongoing project of the Japan Society of Obstetrics, Gynecological and Neonatal Hematology. An intermediate tally has become available from 94 facilities that provided individual survey results, from among 102 facilities where a complete thrombosis survey was completed.

2. A study of the possibility of preventing postoperative obstetric and gynecological DVT by the use of danaparoid sodium (Orgaran).
(1) Subjects: Gynecological surgery (benign, malignant) cases or cesarean section cases, 20 to 75 years of age, at Hamamatsu University School of Medicine. The subjects had given their written consent.
(2) Administration of medication: After confirming the arrest of bleeding within 6 h postoperatively, Orgaran 1250 anti-XaU was given once a day by intravenous injection for 5 days. Control patients received intermittent air massage.
(3) Evaluation: Coagulation-fibrinolysis test preoperatively and at 1, 4, and 7 days postoperatively. Ultrasound Doppler test preoperatively and on the 7th postoperative day.

3. Drafting of guidelines for venous thromboembolism prevention, classified by different risk factors, in obstetrics and gynecology.

Results

Incidence of Obstetrical and Gynecological Thrombosis in Japan

According to an analysis of 94 facilities as of May 2003, in the ongoing survey of the Japan Society of Obstetrics, Gynecological and Neonatal Hematology, the incidence of pulmonary thromboembolism from 1991 to 2000 was 70 cases in obstetrics and 168 cases in gynecology, and is on the increase (Table 1). The incidence in obstetrics consists of 0.02% of total deliveries (70/384,759), 0.006% of vaginal deliveries (17/307,770), and 0.07% of cesarean deliveries (53/76,958); this amounts to 1 case per 5,000 deliveries, which is approaching the level of Western countries. Furthermore, the incidence per cesarean deliveries is 12 times that per vaginal deliveries. The incidence in gynecology, on

TABLE 1. Incidence of pulmonary thromboembolism (PTE) in Japan: analysis of personal data among 94 centers (1991–2000)

Obstetrics: 70 cases, death 7 cases (10%)
Gynecology: 168 cases, death 22 cases (13.1%)
Per total deliveries: 0.02% (70/384,759)
Per vaginal deliveries: 0.006% (17/307,770)
Per total C/S: 0.07% (53/76,989)
Per total operations: 0.08% (168/203,058)
Per benign diseases: 0.03% (51/175,448)
Per malignant diseases: 0.42% (117/27,610)
Fatal rate, 15.4% (18/117)

C/S, cesarean section
Source: Japan Society of Obstetrics, Gynecological and Neonatal Hematology: Kobayashi et al.

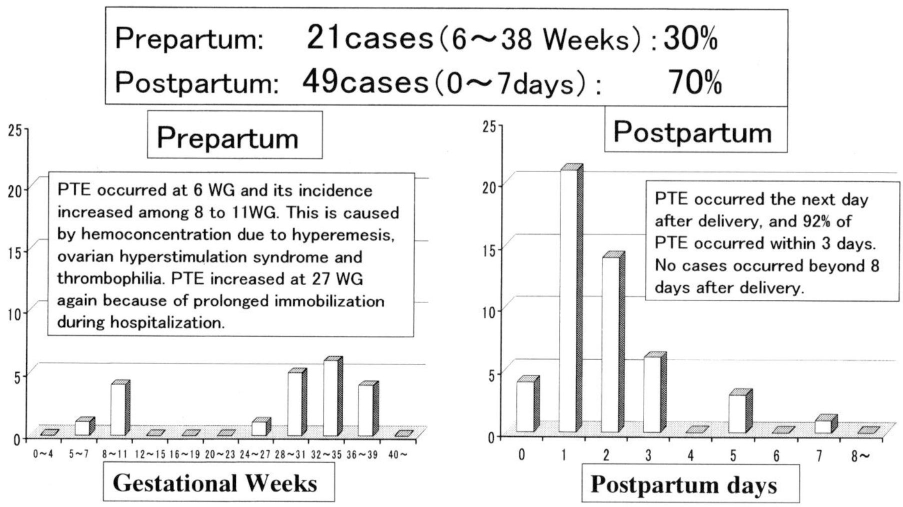

FIG. 1. Occurrence of pulmonary thromboembolism (*PTE*) in obstetrical patients

the other hand, is 0.08% of total operations (168/203,058), 0.03% of benign diseases (51/175,448), and 0.42% of malignant diseases (117/27,610). The incidence in malignant diseases is 14 times that in benign diseases. Malignant diseases included many cases of cancer of the uterine body and ovarian cancer, among whom preoperative PTE was observed, so these patients should be carefully observed preoperatively as well as postoperatively.

Figure 1 shows the different periods of onset of PTE in obstetrical patients: 21 cases, 30%, were prepartum (6–38 weeks), 49 cases, 70%, were postpartum

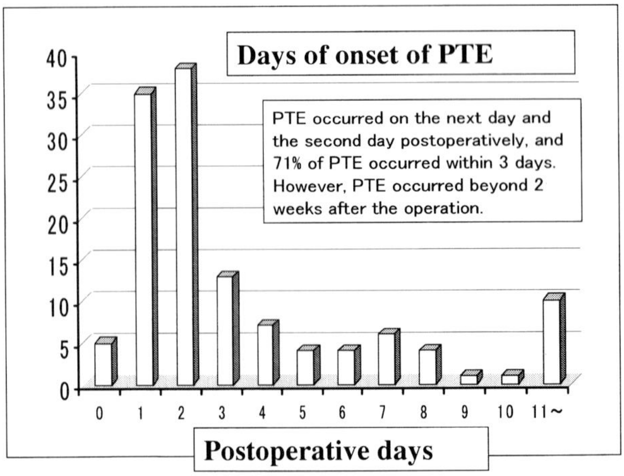

FIG. 2. Occurrence of PTE in gynecological patients

(0–7 days), and the onset appeared in three peaks, at early pregnancy, midterm to late pregnancy, and postpartum. The onset was seen from the 6th gestational week and reached a peak between 8 and 11 weeks. Possible causes are dehydration and immobilization due to hyperemesis, enhanced coagulation and hemoconcentration due to ovarian hyperstimulation syndrome (OHSS), and the onset of thrombophilia in early pregnancy. PTE does not occur after this period, but recurs in midterm and late pregnancy, after 27 gestational weeks, and forms two peaks. This incidence is believed to be caused by prolonged immobilization due to complications of severe preeclampsia, placenta previa, threatened premature labor, and multiple pregnancy. Another large peak was observed postpartum, with the greatest incidence on day 1; 92% of PTE occurred within 3 days postpartum, and all occurred within the first week.

In the occurrence of PTE in gynecological patients (Fig. 2), 27 cases (16.1%) showed preoperative onset. Postoperatively, PTE shows a large peak on days 1 and 2 and subsequently declines, but cases were seen even 2 weeks postoperatively. Gynecological patients, particularly those with malignant disease, need to be observed carefully even after 2 weeks as well as preoperatively.

Changes in Coagulation and Fibrinolytic Factors in Obstetrics and Gynecology

With regard to coagulation and fibrinolytic factors, only changes in D-dimer are presented here. Preoperatively and on postoperative days 1, 4, and 7, changes in D-dimer (μg/ml) in the control groups were 0.6, 2.1, 2.3, and 3.1, respectively, among the benign cases ($n = 44$); 1.9, 7.1, 5.1, and 8.9 among the malignant cases ($n = 8$); and 3.1, 5.8, 5.9, and 4.3 among the cesarean section cases ($n = 9$). All increased significantly postoperatively ($P < 0.01$). In the Orgaran groups the results were, respectively, 0.5, 1.4, 1.3, and 2.0 among the benign cases ($n = 11$); 1.5, 2.3, 3.3, and 6.2 among the malignant cases ($n = 8$); and 3.2, 3.1, 2.7, and 3.5 among the cesarean section cases ($n = 5$). The number was significantly lower ($P < 0.01$) at each postoperative time point compared to the control. DVT onset occurred in cases of cancer of the uterine body in the control group, with markedly high D-dimer changes of 1.1, 9.8, 16.3, and 18.5, respectively.

Drafting of Guidelines for Venous Thromboembolism Prevention, Classified by Different Risk Factors, in Obstetrics and Gynecology

Based on the venous thromboembolism survey of the Japan Society of Obstetrics, Gynecological and Neonatal Hematology, and the results of the study on changes in coagulation and fibrinolytic factors in obstetrics and gynecology, guidelines for the prevention of VTE were drafted (Table 2). First of all, risk groups were placed in four categories of risk—low, moderate; high, highest—similar to the ACCP guidelines. In obstetrics, vaginal delivery was classified as low risk, conventional cesarean section (C/S) delivery as moderate risk, C/S of older or obese patients as high risk, and C/S of cases with a history of VTE or thrombotic factors as highest risk. In gynecology, although the guidelines are based on general abdominal surgery guidelines, the following were identified as specific gynecological risk groups. Namely, a small operation lasting less than 30 min was classified as low risk; benign disease surgery (abdominal, vaginal, laparoscopy), malignant disease surgery that is similar to benign disease surgery, and hormone replacement therapy (HRT) patients as moderate risk; radical surgery for pelvic malignant tumor and benign cases with

TABLE 2. Prevention of perioperative venous thromboembolism (VTE) in obstetrics/gynecology: guidelines according to Japanese evidence of PTE

Risk group	Diseases	Prophylaxis
Low	Small operation, Vaginal delivery	Ambulation
Moderate	Surgery for benign diseases, C/S	ES or IPC
High	C/S + other risks, Radical surgery	IPC or LDUH (±ES)
Highest	High + thrombophilia/DVT	LDUH + IPC or LDUH + ES

Risk should be raised by one rank in case with any additional risks: obesity, age, operation time, blood loss, and other complications

ES, elastic stockings; IPC, intermittent pneumatic compression; LDUH, low-dose unfractionated heparin

a history of VTE or thrombotic factors as high risk; and cases of pelvic malignant tumor with a history of VTE or thrombotic factors as highest risk.

Discussion

In Western nations, the incidence of symptomatic deep venous thrombosis in obstetrical patients is reported to be 0.5 to 7 per 1,000 deliveries, and the number has been decreasing slightly in recent years due to improved prophylaxis [2, 4, 5]. Previously, more than two-thirds of DVT was thought to occur in the puerperal period, particularly in the first week postpartum or the last gestational week, but recent reports describe that DVT can occur at any stage of pregnancy. DVT is five times more prevalent in pregnancy than in nonpregnant periods, and occurs seven- to tenfold more frequently in C/S compared to vaginal deliveries [1, 5–8]. Approximately 4% to 5% of obstetrical DVT could lead to pulmonary thromboembolism, and, conversely, more than 90% of pulmonary thromboembolism cases are thought to be caused by DVT of the lower extremities [9]. Once PTE occurs it is extremely serious, with a mortality rate reported to be 18% to 30% [10] if left untreated, and has long been the leading cause of maternal mortalities [1, 11, 12]. In Japan as well, according to maternal and child health statistics of Japan, the percentage of obstetrical PTE, including amniotic fluid embolism, in the maternal mortality rate was 23.5% (20/85) in 1995 and 22.4% (17/76) in 2001, making it the leading cause of direct obstetrical deaths (Fig. 3) [13]. Furthermore, most PTE cases occur in the puerperal period, and the majority of those cases occur after C/S [5, 14, 15].

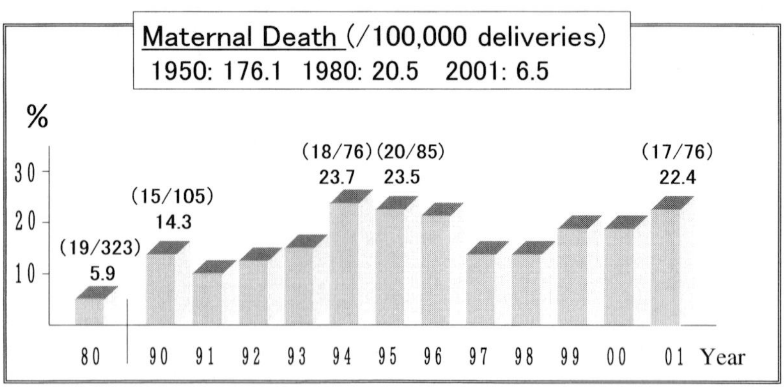

Fig. 3. Incidence of obstetrical PTE (including amniotic fluid embolism) in the rate of maternal deaths in Japan

There are few reports regarding the incidence of DVT in the gynecology field. According to research conducted by Nicolaides et al. using the ^{125}I-fibrinogen uptake test, the incidence of DVT after general surgery was 40.3% (133/330), of which 45% occurred on the day of the operation [16]. In Japan, Matsumoto et al. conducted a similar study and found that the incidence of postoperative DVT was 10.8% (7/65) in all gynecological surgery and 19.4% (6/31) in radical hysterectomy or modified radical hysterectomy [17], which may be a lower rate than in the West but is not by any means a small figure. Furthermore, statistics from Keio University Obstetrics & Gynecology Department confirmed that the incidence of postoperative symptomatic PTE was 26 (0.8%) among 3,203 gynecological surgery cases (excluding pregnancy-related operations) in a 5-year period, 1993–1997, and that the incidence was increasing annually. Gynecological surgery involves pelvic procedures in many cases and thus has a higher rate of VTE than in general surgery. Particularly in the case of radical hysterectomy or modified radical hysterectomy with accompanying lymph node resection, symptomatic PTE reached 3.8%, and cases that required paraaortic lymph node resection had an incidence of 7.8% [18].

According to Nicolaides et al., the incidence of postoperative DVT, including asymptomatic cases, is less than 1% to 10% in small operations of short duration, 10% to 40% in moderate-risk patients over 40 years of age, and is believed to be 40% to 80% in high-risk patients with a history of VTE or malignant tumor patients requiring extended surgery. Furthermore, the incidence of fatal PTE is reported to be less than 0.01%, 0.1% to 0.8%, and 1% to 5%, respectively; Japanese data of this kind are currently not available [19].

In the West, particularly among Caucasians, there is a prevalence of thrombosis caused by genetic structural abnormalities of clotting factors, which is further aggravated by environmental factors to produce a high rate of VTE. Because the Japanese ethnically have fewer structural abnormalities of clotting factors, environmental factors, pregnancy and labor, and invasive surgery play a major role in the occurrence of VTE [1, 15].

As our survey has clarified, VTE has been on the rise in Japan in recent years, together with the Westernization of our eating habits. In the field of obstetrics and gynecology as well, VTE has been increasing steadily, and preventive measures are urgently needed. Prevention of deep venous thrombosis is associated with the prevention of pulmonary thromboembolism and, therefore, when there are risk factors in the perinatal period, the following measures should be taken postpartum [1, 2, 9, 14, 17, 18]. Even in vaginal delivery cases, which are low risk, early ambulation is recommended.

1. General prophylaxis: early ambulation, leg elevation in bed, and exercises such as bending/stretching the knees and dorsal flexion of the legs,

wearing elastic stockings (ES), intermittent pneumatic compression (IPC), and prevention of dehydration are recommended for general prophylaxis. In C/S cases, it is better to have the patient in the dorsal position and to avoid the lithotomy position.

2. Prophylaxis by medication

a. Low-dose unfractionated heparin: 5000 units b.i.d. by subcutaneous injection within 6–12 h postoperatively (or immediately postoperatively if the arrest of bleeding is confirmed), to be administered for 3–5 days.

b. Warfarin: The target is a thrombotest result of 30% (PT-INR 1.5–2.0). If the risk is high, continue administration for 1–3 months after heparin treatment.

Heparin is not considered to be transferable to the fetus or to the infant via breast milk. With regard to warfarin the reports vary, but most agree that there is no transition through breast milk. In any case, it is advisable to give the infant vitamin K syrup to prevent vitamin K deficiency bleeding disorder.

Prophylactic heparin therapy is recommended for postoperative C/S patients who have risk factors. Conventional heparin, however, has the side effect of hemorrhage and is generally avoided for postoperative use. Low molecular weight heparin, which is less likely to cause bleeding, is therefore used in the West. Because low molecular weight heparin has not yet been approved in Japan, we are using low-dose unfractionated heparin for prophylaxis, after confirming the arrest of bleeding 6–12h postoperatively.

Compared to low-dose unfractionated heparin, low molecular weight heparin has a lower prevalence of side effects in addition to hemorrhage, such as heparin-induced thrombocytopenia (HIT), allergic reaction, and osteoporosis, and furthermore requires less blood coagulation monitoring; it is therefore used routinely in Western countries. In Japan, however, low molecular weight heparin is not covered by health insurance and is contraindicated for pregnant women.

Danaparoid sodium is a low molecular weight heparinoid, with heparin sulfate as its main component, and is a selective Xa factor inhibitor, as is low molecular weight heparin. It has fewer side effects than low-dose unfractionated heparin and can be administered to pregnant women, but it is not covered by insurance for the indication of venous thromboembolism.

When using a drug that does not have the indication of venous thromboembolism prevention, as described above, sufficient informed consent is needed. Also, we should exercise caution in the postoperative use of antifibrinolytic agents such as tranexamic acid.

Furthermore, users of oral contraceptives have a higher risk of VTE compared to nonusers. To prevent VTE in women in general as well as women scheduled for an operation, we should (1) avoid administration of oral contraceptives to women with a high risk of VTE and (2) conduct blood coagulation tests if the possibility of VTE onset is suspected, avoiding administration if there are any abnormalities. We should always be on the alert for early signs of VTE.

Based on the results of the study on the prevention of deep venous thrombosis in obstetrics and gynecology using danaparoid sodium, the following could be considered as a guide to postoperative thrombosis prevention: (1) for patients with benign disease, early mobilization and massage are sufficient and anticoagulant therapy is unnecessary if there are no other risk factors; (2) for C/S patients in whom enhanced coagulation is evident preoperatively and continues postoperatively, if anticoagulant therapy is administered, less than 5 days is sufficient as the coagulation will be suppressed within a week; (3) for patients with malignant disease with marked postoperative coagulation that continues after a week has elapsed, if anticoagulant therapy is administered it should be for more than 1 week; and (4) D-dimer analysis has been found to be a useful predictor of postoperative thrombosis. It seems highly probable that thrombosis will increase in the future, and its prevention is of the utmost importance.

Prospective studies must be carried out in addition to retrospective studies to elucidate risk factors in the Japanese population. We need to conduct many clinical trials to establish VTE prevention guidelines that are suited to Japanese patients.

Last, let me stress the need to have the patient and her family be aware of the risk of VTE. For this objective, we should place pamphlets about VTE in the waiting room and make sure the patient is given a full explanation. When heparin is administered for prophylactic purposes, it is advisable to obtain the patient's written consent. Furthermore, in case of an emergency it is important to maintain close contact with the patient's family.

References

1. Kobayashi T. Pulmonary thromboembolism. In: Taketani Y, Aono T, Aso T, et al., editors. Comprehensive handbook of women's medicine. Vol. 8 (in Japanese). Tokyo: Nakayama-Shoten; 1999. p. 249–62.
2. Bates SM, Ginsberg JS. Thrombosis in pregnancy. Curr Opin Haematol 1997;4:335–43.
3. Kobayashi T. Deep venous thromboembolism: incidence in obstetrical and gynecological field (in Japanese). Curr Ther 2002;20(4):347–50.
4. Bergqvist A, Bergqvist D, Hallbook T. Thrombosis during pregnancy: a prospective study. Acta Obstet Gynecol Scand 1983;62:443–8.
5. Rutherford S, Montoro M, McGehee W, et al. Thromboembolic disease associated with pregnancy: an 11 year review (abstract). Am J Obstet Gynecol 1991;164(suppl): 286.

6. Tengborn L, Berqvist D, Matzch T, et al. Recurrent thromboembolism in pregnancy and puerperium: is there a need for thromboprophylaxis? Am J Obstet Gynecol 1989;160:90–4.
7. Ginsberg JS, Brill-Edwards P, Burrows RF, et al. Venous thrombosis during pregnancy: leg and trimester of presentation. Thromb Haemostasis 1992;67:519–20.
8. Sugimura M, Ohashi R, Itakura S, et al. Pulmonary thromboembolism in obstetrical and gynecological field (in Japanese). Jpn J Thromb Hemost 2001;12:460–66.
9. Baker WF. Diagnosis of deep vein thrombosis and pulmonary embolism. Med Clin N Am 1998;82:459–76.
10. Kemp PM, Tarver D, Batty V, et al. Pulmonary embolism: is the clinical history a useful adjunct to aid interpretation of the equivocal lung scan? Clin Nucl Med 1996;21:203–7.
11. Kaunitz AM, Hughes JM, Grimes DA, et al. Causes of maternal mortality in the United States. Obstet Gynecol 1985;65:605–12.
12. Atrash HK, Koonin LM, Lawson HW, et al. Maternal mortality in the United States: 1979 $< n <$ 1986. Obstet Gynecol 1990;76:1055–60.
13. Mothers' & Children's Health & Welfare Association. Maternal and child health statistics of Japan (in Japanese). Tokyo, Mothers' & Children's Health Organization, 2003. p. 76–8.
14. Kobayashi T. Acute pulmonary thromboembolism in Japan. Obstetrical and gynecological field. Ther Res 2003;24(4):613–5 (in Japanese).
15. Terao T. Thrombophilia in obstetrical and gynecological field. Jpn J Obstet Gynecol Neonatal Hematol 1996;6:12–32 (in Japanese).
16. Nicolaides AN, Gordan-Smith L. A rational approach to prevention. In: Nicolaides AN, editor. Thromboembolism, aetiology, advances in prevention and management. Lancaster, Medical and Technical Publishing, 1975.
17. Matsumoto K, Hirose H, Hayashi K, et al. Study on postoperative venous thrombosis. Jpn J Phlebol 1994;5:163–9 (in Japanese).
18. Aoki D. Postoperative pulmonary thromboembolism in gynecological surgery. Kanto J Obstet Gynecol 1998;35:284 (abstract, in Japanese).
19. Nicolaides AN, Bergqvist D, Hull RD, et al. Prevention of venous thromboembolism. International consensus statement. Int Angiol 1997;16:3–38.

Prevention and Treatment of Thrombosis in Pregnancy: The Newest Treatment Approaches

Sheri Lynn Hamersley

Introduction

Thromboembolic disease remains the leading cause of nonobstetric maternal mortality in the United States [1]. Moreover, recent studies have evaluated not only the potential maternal complications, but also fetal risks. The morbidity and mortality results from thrombosis can be drastically reduced by testing, and possibly treating, those patients at risk. It can also be reduced by identifying and treating symptomatic women with a strong clinical suspicion for deep venous thrombosis (DVT) and/or pulmonary embolism (PE). The difficulty lies in the risk of overtreatment versus undertreatment.

Epidemiology

The risk of thrombosis in pregnancy increased tenfold when compared with age-matched controls [2]. This risk is higher after cesarean section than vaginal delivery [3]. The recurrence rate of thrombosis during pregnancy with a prior history of a venous thromboembolic event (VTE) is 0% to 13% [4]. The recurrence risk for patients with abnormal test results and a previous episode of VTE is 5.9% [5]. Asymptomatic women with congenital deficiencies have an eightfold risk of VTE, compared with normal control subjects [6]. One study revealed that 60% of women who develop VTE during pregnancy have a factor V Leiden mutation [7]. Until recently, there were no reliable studies to evaluate the true incidence of recurrent VTE in pregnant women with a prior history of thrombosis.

In 2000, Brill-Edwards and Ginsberg completed a prospective study that was published in the *New England Journal of Medicine* [8]. They evaluated 125

15005 Shady Grove Road Ste 340, Rockville, MD 20850, USA

pregnant women with a single episode of objectively diagnosed VTE and withheld their antepartum heparin. Warfarin was given 4 to 6 weeks postpartum with a targeted international normalized ratio (INR) of 2.0 to 3.0 followed by either unfractionated heparin (UH) or low molecular weight heparin (LMWH). The recurrence rate was 2.4% unless a thrombophilia was identified, in which case the rate was 5.9%. In the 44 patients without an identified thrombophilia, there were no recurrences. The conclusion based on these results was that the absolute risk of antepartum recurrent VTE is women without thrombophilia is low and antepartum heparin is not routinely justified [9]. This study, however, did not address the potential fetal complications as it focused only on the maternal risk of recurrent VTE.

Pathophysiology

Virchow described a triad of risk factors for VTE over 140 years ago that included venous stasis, vessel wall damage, and hypercoagulability. VTE is now generally considered a multifactorial disorder, with interactions between genetic, acquired, and environmental risk factors [10]. There are many changes that occur in pregnancy that predispose the normal female to VTE. Venous distension begins in the first trimester, and venous flow to the lower extremities is reduced by half by the third trimester. There is also an increase in all clotting factors, except factors XI and XIII. Fibrinolytic inhibitors may be produced by the placenta. Protein S levels decrease by about 10% in the first trimester of normal pregnancies. Moreover, if a patient is carrying a multiple gestation or if she is required to undergo complete bed rest, then the risks are compounded. Other predisposing factors include advanced maternal age, obesity, smoking, and cesarean delivery.

Thrombophilias

Thrombophilias, or an increased propensity toward clotting, can be classified as either hereditary or acquired. Examples of hereditary thrombophilias associated with adverse pregnancy outcomes include protein S and C deficiency, antithrombin II deficiency, factor V Q506 mutation (Leiden), prothrombin 20210A mutation, and methylene tetrahydrofolate reductase deficiency (MTHFR)/hyperhomocysteinemia (Table 1).

Free protein S acts as a cofactor with anticoagulant protein C to inactivate clotting factors Va and VIIa (Fig. 1).

Protein S deficiency has autosomal dominant inheritance and, therefore, offspring should be considered for testing by a pediatric hematologist. The risk for VTE in heterozygous carriers is 1% to 3%. Protein C inactivates factors

TABLE 1. Hereditary thrombophilias

Protein S deficiency
Protein C deficiency
Antithrombin III deficiency
Factor V Q506 mutation (Leiden)
Prothrombin 20210A mutation
Methylene tetrahydrofolate reductase deficiency (MTHFR)/ hyperhomocysteinemia

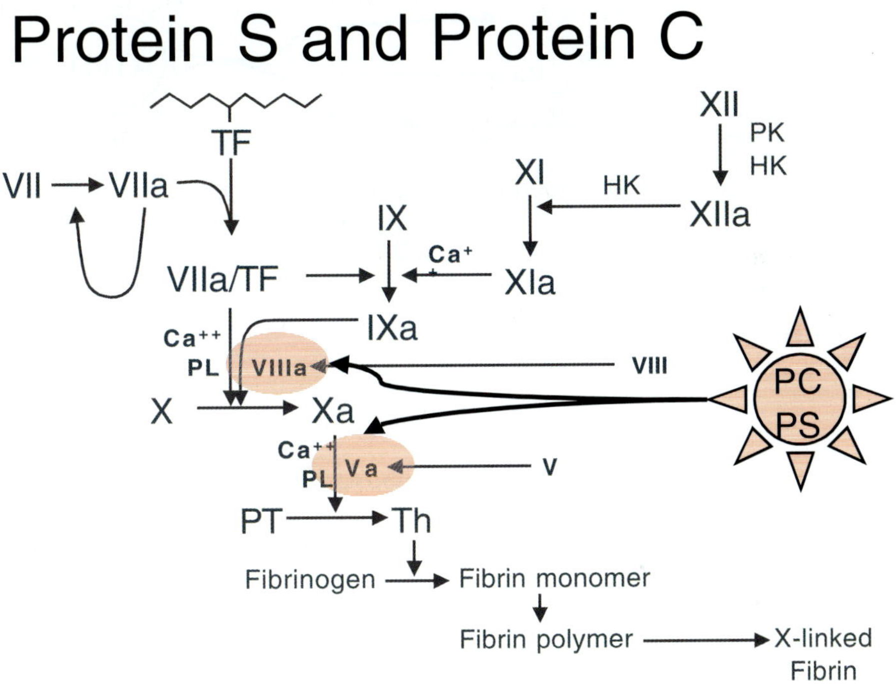

FIG. 1. Intrinsic and extrinsic pathways

Va and VIIIa and is inherited in an autosomal dominant fashion with incomplete penetrance. The prevalence in the general pregnant population is 0.5%, and the risk for VTE in affected patients is 1% to 3.1%.

Antithrombin inactivates thrombin and factors Xa, Ixa, and XIIa. It is inherited in an autosomal dominant manner. There is a 40% to 70% risk of developing VTE with an antithrombin III deficiency (Fig. 2).

Factor V Leiden mutation is associated with an activated protein C resistance and is the most common genetic defect resulting in thrombosis with a

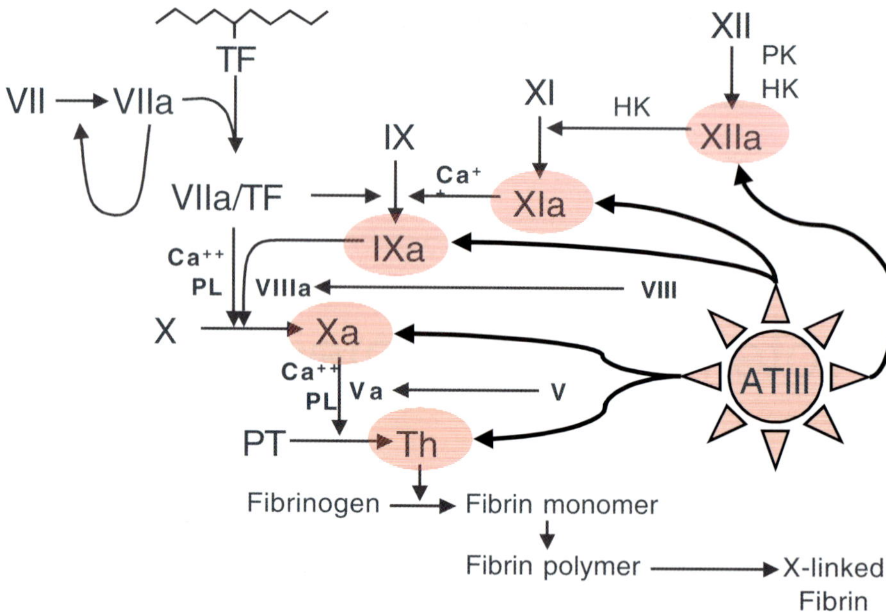

FIG. 2. Antithrombin III

prevalence of 5% to 7%. The risk of thrombosis with this defect is 0.5%. The prothrombin mutation (20210A) has a prevalence of 2% and a 0.5% risk of VTE associated with its presence.

Methylene tetrahydrafolate reductase (MTHFR) is important in folate synthesis and folic acid is necessary in the methylation of homocysteine. An MTHFR mutation can predispose an individual to hyperhomocysteinemia and thus increase risk for thrombosis.

Homozygous mutations (two copies of the mutation) may be associated with increased risk for offspring to develop open neural tube defects (ONTD) such as spina bifida. Acquired thrombophilias include antiphospholipid antibody syndrome (APLS) and anticardiolipin antibodies (ACA) (Table 2). Antiphospholipid-mediated thrombosis results from interference with phospholipid-associated anticoagulant proteins [e.g., beta 2 glycoprotein 1 (B2GP1), antithrobin III, annexin V, protein C, and protein S].

Anticardiolipin antibodies and lupus anticoagulant (LAC) are the most common acquired causes of thrombophilia and adverse perinatal outcome (Table 3). The prevalence is 9% to 14% associated with a first episode of VTE, and there is a 20% to 50% recurrence risk for thrombosis. Antiphospholipid

TABLE 2. Acquired thrombophilias

Antiphospholipid antibody syndrome (APLS)
Anticardiolipin antibodies (ACA)
Lupus anticoagulant (LAC)

TABLE 3. Criteria for diagnosis of APLS*

APLS	
Clinical	Serological
Venous thrombosis	ACA IgG 20-80GPL
Arterial thrombosis	IgM 20-MPL
Recurrent Pregnancy loss	
Thrombocytopenia	Positive LAC aPTT
	dRVVT, platelet neutraliz

*Patients with one clinical + one serologic feature

antibodies are associated with autoimmune disorders such as lupus, infectious organisms such as Lyme, and medications such as procainamide, oral contraceptives, dilantin, and chlorpromazine.

Two main adverse experiences associated with thrombophilias in pregnancy include venous thromboembolic phenomenon and pregnancy complications. Commonly associated pregnancy complications include placental infarction, recurrent miscarriage, intrauterine growth restriction (IUGR), severe preeclampsia, abruption, and intrauterine fetal demise (IUFD).

Treatment and Prevention

The treatment and prevention of VTE in pregnancy revolves around the use of anticoagulants: these include unfractionated heparins (UH), low molecular weight heparins (LMWH), warfarin (coumadin), and/or aspirin.

Unfractionated heparins are naturally occurring mucopolysaccarides that bind to antithrombin III to inhibit thrombin. They also increase levels of activated factor X (Xa) inhibitor. They are usually fairly large molecules (average 15,000 daltons); however, they do not cross the placental barrier as they are highly charged. They are also rapidly reversed with protamine sulfate. Potential side effects include IgG-mediated thrombocytopenia, osteoporosis, and bleeding.

LMWH is a Category B drug (extremely safe in pregnancy) and has an average molecular weight of 5,000 daltons. These substances inhibit factor Xa,

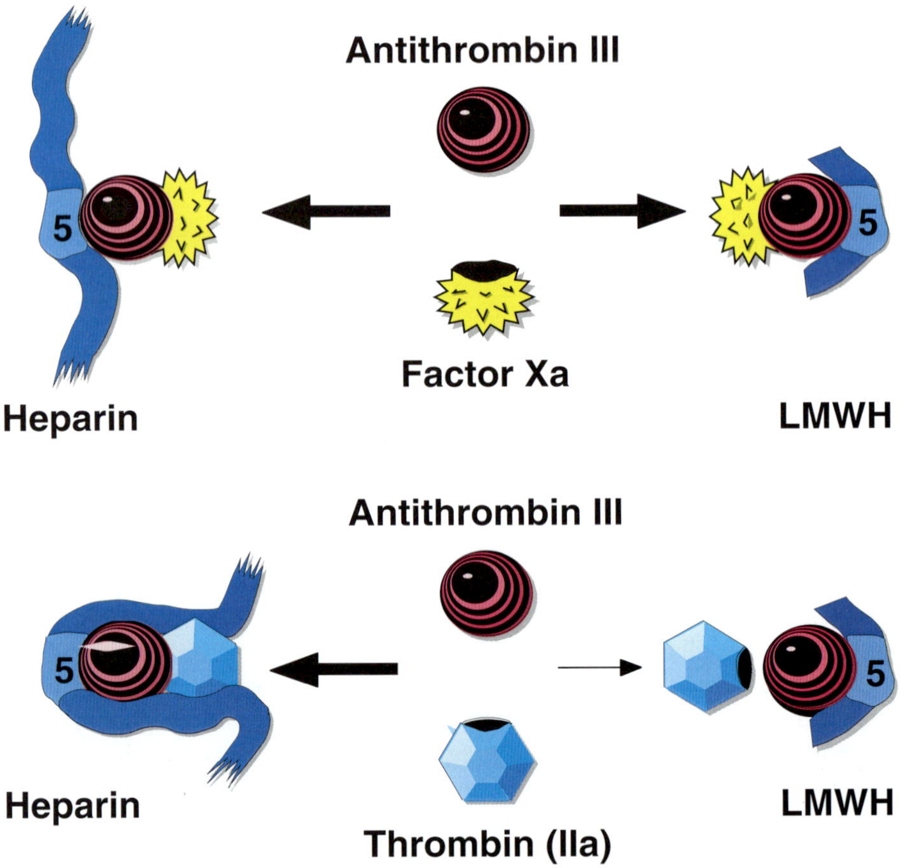

FIG. 3. Low molecular weight heparins (*LMWH*) versus unfractionated heparins (UH)

but not thrombin, and therefore cause less bleeding than UH. They have a low affinity for plasma proteins and a more consistent bioavailability. They have a longer (4h) half-life than UH (3h) and are less likely to be associated with heparin-induced thrombocytopenia or osteoporosis (Fig. 3).

Warfarin

Warfarin, or coumadin, inhibits regeneration of vitamin K dependent clotting factors and easily crosses the placenta. Its use in the first trimester has been associated with nasal hypoplasia, depression of the nasal bridge, and there is a 30% incidence of developmental delay. It has also been associated with central nervous system abnormalities and fetal hemorrhage. These findings have collectively been referred to as "the Warfarin syndrome."

Low-Dose Aspirin

Low-dose aspirin (81 mg/day) has been shown to have an antiplatelet effect and to enhance the leukocyte-derived interleukin-3 (IL-3) production. IL-3 is a cytokine that has been shown to stimulate placental growth.

Treatment of Deep Venous Thrombosis and Pulmonary Thrombosis

There are two alternative approaches: intravenous unfractionated heparin (UFH) followed by at least 3 months of subcutaneous heparin with dose-adjusted partial thromboplastin time, or subcutaneous low molecular weight heparin (LMWH) used for both initial and long-term treatment.

Prevention of Venous Thromboembolism: Categorized

Single episode VTE; transient risk factor
Single episode VTE and thrombophilia
No prior VTE and thrombophilia
Multiple (2 or more) episodes
VTE; receiving long-term anticoagulation.

Prevention of Venous Thromboembolism

Two general approaches for the prevention of VTE are active prophylaxis with UFH or LMWH or clinical surveillance. Preventive doses of LMWH are targeted to an anti-Xa peak level of 0.2 to 0.6 U/ml [30–40 mg subcutaneously (sq) bid]. UFH at 5,000 sq bid in the first trimester, 7,500 bid in the second trimester, and 10,000 bid in the third trimester is generally a good rule of thumb.

Prosthetic Heart Valve Patients

Patients with prosthetic heart valves have a high maternal mortality (2.9%). These patients require higher doses of UFH (17,500–20,000 units q12 h) or LMWH (setting the anti-Xa level at about 1.5 U/ml) to fully anticoagulate and low-dose aspirin. The use of warfarin in these patients is associated with a 6.4% risk of embryopathy.

Conclusions and Recommendations

Pregnant women are at increased risk for thromboembolic disease, which is the leading cause of maternal mortality. Some predisposing conditions may increase this risk even further. Anticoagulation therapy is indicated during pregnancy for the prevention and treatment of VTE.

Patients with recurrent pregnancy loss, severe intrauterine growth restriction (IUGR), severe pregnancy induced hypertension (PIH), or VTE should warrant testing for thrombophilias. Women who are homozygous for the MTHFR mutation should be treated with folic acid supplements before and during pregnancy. Women with a thrombophilic deficit and recurrent miscarriages should be considered for low-dose aspirin and possibly LMWH.

Low molecular weight heparins are safe in pregnancy, and are associated with fewer potential side effects when compared with UH.

References

1. Sachs BP, Brown DA, Driscoll SG, et al. Maternal mortality in Massachusetts: trends and prevention. N Engl J Med 1987;316:607–72.
2. Bonnar J. Venous thromboembolism and pregnancy. Clin Obstet Gynecol 1981; 8(2):455–73.
3. Greer IA. Thrombosis in pregnancy: maternal and fetal issues. Lancet 1999; 353:1258–65.
4. Tengborn L. Recurrent thromboembolism in pregnancy and puerperium: is there a need for thromboprophylaxis? Am J Obstet Gynecol 1989;160:90–4.
5. Ginsberg JS. Thromboembolism and pregnancy. Thromb Haemostasis 1999;82(2): 620–5.
6. Friederich PW, Sanson BJ, Simioni P, et al. Frequency of pregnancy-related venous thromboembolism in anticoagulant factor-deficient women: implications for prophylaxis. Arch Intern Med 1996;125:955–60.
7. Hellgren M, Svensson PJ, Dalback B. Resistance to activated protein C as a basis for VTE associated with pregnancy and oral contraceptives. Am J Obstet Gynecol 1995;173:210–13.
8. Brill-Edwards P, Ginsberg J, Gent M, et al. Safety of withholding heparin in pregnant women with a history of VTE. N Engl J Med 2000;343:1439–44.
9. Middledorp S, Henkens CMA, Koopman MMW, et al. The incidence of venous thromboembolism in women who are homozygous for factor V Leiden. Br J Haematol 2001;113:553–5.
10. Kupferminc M, Amiram E, et al. Increased frequency of genetic thrombophilia in women with complications of pregnancy. N Engl J Med 1999;340(1):9–13.

Thromboprophylaxis in the Cancer Patient

Ajay K. Kakkar

Introduction

It has long been recognized that thrombosis is associated with malignant disease [1]. In his original description, Trousseau links the occurrence of a spontaneous thrombophlebitis with the presence of underlying malignant disease. Patients with established cancer are also at greater risk for the development of thromboembolic disease secondary to the malignancy itself, part of the intervention they are receiving for treatment of their cancer, and the debilitation and immobility associated with the advancing stage of their disease.

The hypercoagulable state is often recognized in patients with malignant disease. This condition appears to be secondary to tumor elaboration of the physiological initiator of blood coagulation tissue factor [2]. Patients with solid tumor malignancy have higher circulating levels of tissue factor associated with a marked elevation in levels of factor VIIa, indicating extrinsic pathway activation. They also have evidence of excessive systemic thrombin generation [3].

Cancer Interventions

Although it is recognized that thrombosis may complicate the course of a number of different cancers, the impact of tumor type on the frequency of thromboembolic complications is poorly understood. The clinical manifestation of venous thromboembolism in the cancer patient extends from asymptomatic distal deep vein thrombosis to fatal pulmonary embolism.

Centre for Surgical Sciences, Barts and The London School for Medicine and Dentistry, and Thrombosis Research Institute, Emmanuel Kaye Building, Manresa Road, London SW3 6LR, UK

Kakkar et al. in 1970 demonstrated that cancer patients undergoing surgical intervention had a higher risk for the development of deep vein thrombosis compared to noncancer patients [3]. Since that time, numerous other studies have confirmed these original findings and have also demonstrated that fatal pulmonary embolism after major surgery in cancer patients is significantly higher that in noncancer patients (1.6% vs. 0.4%) [4]. Evidence suggests that in patients with malignant disease venous thromboembolism is the second most common cause of death [5, 6]. Overall, some 15% of cancer patients will experience symptomatic thromboembolic disease during the course of their disease [7–9].

There have been more limited studies that have assessed the risk of thromboembolic complications associated with chemotherapeutic intervention. The best investigated population of patients are women with breast cancer receiving either adjuvant or palliative chemotherapy. In a study of postmenopausal women receiving adjuvant therapy for breast cancer, the combination of Tamoxifen with cytotoxic chemotherapy was associated with an increase in risk from 1.4% for Tamoxifen alone to 9.6% for the combination ($P = 0.0001$) [8]. Cancer patients receiving cytotoxic chemotherapy for management of breast cancer appear to be at greatest risk for the development of thrombosis while they are actively receiving their anticancer treatment [9]. Beyond the use of chemotherapy, intervention with radiotherapy also appears to increase the risk of thrombosis in certain cancer populations. For instance, in patients with rectal cancer receiving neoadjuvant radiotherapy, there is an increase in risk for the development of subsequent postoperative venous thromboembolism from 3.6% to 7.5% ($P = 0.001$) [10].

Prevention of Venous Thromboembolic Disease in Cancer Surgical Patients

The frequency of thromboembolic complications in cancer patients is of sufficient magnitude, and the consequences in terms of symptomatic thrombosis and fatal pulmonary embolism in particular are so devastating, that mandatory thromboprophylaxis is recognized to be essential in cancer patients undergoing major surgical intervention.

A number of methods are available including mechanical and pharmacological approaches. In terms of mechanical methods of prevention of thromboembolic disease in cancer patients, there is limited evidence for their benefit. Small studies have indicated that intermittent compression of the calf can reduce the frequency of postoperative deep vein thrombosis from 21% to 12% [11]. However, this form of prophylaxis has never been demonstrated to be effective in reducing the frequency of pulmonary embolism in cancer patients.

Pharmacological methods such as aspirin and dextran have not been adequately assessed in cancer patients, and no recommendation can be made about their use in this population.

Unfractionated low-dose subcutaneous heparin has been extensively evaluated for the prevention of thromboembolic disease in high-risk surgical populations. In a meta-analysis of low-dose heparin studies in which its efficacy was compared against controls or placebo, data from 919 patients with cancer demonstrated that low-dose unfractionated heparin, administered perioperatively, reduced the frequency of postoperative deep vein thrombosis from 30.6% in the control group to 13.6% in the heparin group ($P = 0.001$) [12]. Low-dose unfractionated heparin has also been shown to reduce the frequency of fatal pulmonary embolism in high-risk surgical patients, including those with malignant disease [13].

More recently, the low molecular weight heparins have replaced low-dose unfractionated heparin. The benefits of low molecular weight heparins include a more predictable bioavailability after subcutaneous administration, a longer plasma half-life, and a lower frequency of thrombocytopenia and osteoporosis when compared to unfractionated heparin. It is for this reason that low molecular weight heparins have replaced low-dose unfractionated heparin for thromboprophylaxis. Low molecular weight heparins have been extensively investigated for thromboprophylaxis for a large number of surgical patients. However, there are very few studies that have specifically investigated their benefit for venous thromboembolism prophylaxis in patients with cancer. Bergqvist et al. [14] randomized more than 2000 patients, 65% of whom were undergoing operation for malignant disease, to receive prophylaxis with a standard- or higher-risk prophylactic dose of low molecular weight heparin (Dalteparin). He was able to demonstrate that increasing the dose of perioperative low molecular weight heparin reduced the frequency of postoperative deep vein thrombosis from 14.9% in the standard-dose group to 8.5% in the higher-dose group, without any significant increase in bleeding complications.

Further data about the safety of low molecular weight heparins in cancer surgical patients have been provided by studies in neurosurgical patients, many of whom have undergone operations for intracranial malignancy. In a study of some 300 patients [15], many of whom were undergoing operation for intracranial malignancy, patients were randomized to receive low molecular weight heparin or placebo in combination with graduated lower limb compression stockings. The addition of low molecular weight heparin reduced the frequency of postoperative thromboembolic complications in this high-risk group without any significant increase in bleeding complications.

More recently, dermatan sulfate (glycosaminoglycan), which inhibits heparin cofactor II and thus achieves a antithrombotic effect, has been assessed in more than 800 patients randomized to receive this agent or low-dose unfractionated heparin. The patients were undergoing operation for cancer. The frequency of deep vein thrombosis in the heparin group was 22%, reduced to 15% in that group of patients receiving dermatan sulfate [16].

The duration of thromboprophylaxis has recently been assessed in canscer surgical patients. Current recommendations indicate the patients undergoing operation for malignant disease should receive at least 7 to 10 days of thromboprophylaxis with low-dose or low molecular weight heparin while in the hospital. A recent study randomized patients at the time of hospital discharge to continue with placebo or low molecular weight heparin for a further 3 weeks with venographic screening for thrombosis at the end of this period. The frequency of deep vein thrombosis was reduced from 12% in the group of patients who received prophylaxis in hospital to only 4% when prophylaxis was continued into the postdischarge period [17].

Thromboprophylaxis in Nonsurgical Cancer Patients

There are many fewer data available in the published literature with regard to the efficacy and safety of routine thromboprophylactic intervention in nonsurgical cancer patients. Only one randomized trial has assessed the benefits of such intervention in women with advanced breast cancer receiving cytotoxic chemotherapy. In this trial, more than 300 women receiving chemotherapy were randomized to low-dose Warfarin or placebo. The international normalized ratio was maintained at between 1.3 and 1.9 in the Warfarin group. The frequency of thrombotic complications was reduced by 85%, from 4.4% in the control group to 0.6% in the Warfarin group ($P = 0.003$) [18].

Another group of patients who have historically been considered to be at high risk for the development of thromboembolic complications are cancer patients with indwelling central venous catheters. Two studies in the early 1990s [19, 20] evaluated 1 mg Warfarin or 2500 units low molecular weight heparin Dalteparin, respectively, in the prevention of central venous catheter-associated thrombosis. In the first study, with Warfarin rates of thrombosis were reduced from 37% to 9% when screened using upper limb venography [19]. In the second study, rates of thrombosis were reduced from more than 60% to 6% with the use of Dalteparin [20]. However, contemporary studies assessing the value of these interventions in patients receiving modern central venous catheters suggest that the rates of thrombosis are now much lower, and it is difficult at this stage to recommend routine antithrombotic therapy in this population.

Low Molecular Weight Heparin Therapy in Survival in Cancer

An intriguing recent observation has been that chronic administration of low molecular weight heparin may be associated with enhanced survival in cancer patients. A meta-analysis of deep vein thrombosis treatment studies undertaken in the early 1990s suggested that cancer patients who received low molecular weight heparin for initial treatment of their deep vein thrombosis had a lower mortality after 3 months than those who received intravenous unfractionated heparin [21, 22].

Recently, the Fragmin Advance Malignancy Outcome Study (FAMOUS), the first prospective randomized placebo-controlled trial, has assessed the value of up to 1 year of low molecular weight heparin therapy with Dalteparin sodium in patients with advanced malignant disease [23]. Three hundred and eighty-five patients with advanced cancer were randomized to receive Dalteparin in a dose of 5000 units or placebo injection. The study failed to detect a significant difference in overall survival between the two populations. However, in a subgroup of patients, identified post hoc, there was an increase in median survival from 23 to 43 months in favour of Dalteparin.

In a further study of 302 patients who were randomized to receive either low molecular weight heparin for 6 weeks or placebo [24], those receiving the low molecular weight heparin Nandroparin demonstrated a significant survival advantage at up to 84 months of follow-up. Similarly, in a trial of 84 patients with small cell lung cancer [25] who were all receiving chemotherapy but were additionally randomized to receive the low molecular weight heparin Dalteparin or no antithrombotic therapy, there was an increase in both overall survival and disease-free survival for those patients with lung cancer receiving the low molecular weight heparin.

Although the mechanism for these apparent survival benefits associated with the low molecular weight heparin treatment in cancer patients remains unclear, further trials are warranted to investigate their potential benefit.

Conclusions

Thrombosis is an important complication in cancer patients. Cancer surgical patients receiving thromboprophylaxis with either low-dose or low molecular weight heparin are protected against thrombosis, this intervention has been validated in terms of efficacy and safety. In non-surgical cancer patients, those with breast cancer may receive low-dose oral anticoagulation with vitamin K antagonists. The benefit of routine thromboprophylaxis in other ambulant cancer populations receiving medical therapy for their cancers remains to be established by way of prospective clinical trials. For cancer patients with central venous catheters, no recommendations can be made about routine antithrombotic therapy, although certain patients at high risk could be considered for either vitamin K antagonists (Warfarin, 1 mg) or low molecular weight heparin (Dalteparin, 2500 units). The intriguing observation that low molecular weight heparin therapy may be associated with enhanced survival has become more plausible with the evidence generated from contemporary prospective clinical trials. However, further clinical trials in specific cancer populations are required before low molecular weight heparins may be used for this exciting indication.

References

1. Plegmasia alba dolens. In: Trousseau A. Lectures on clinical medicine (delivered at the Hotel-Dieu, Paris, France). Cormack JR, trans. London: The New Syndeham Society, 1872:282–332.
2. Kakkar AK, DeRuvo N, Chinswangwatanakul V, et al. Extrinsic-pathway activation in cancer with high factor VIIa and tissue factor. Lancet 1995;346(8981):1004–5.
3. Kakkar VV, Howe CT, Nicolaides AN, et al. Deep vein thrombosis of the leg. Is there a "high risk" group? Am J Surg 1970;120:527–30.
4. Rahr HB, Sorensen JV. Venous thromboembolism and cancer. Blood Coagul Fibrinolysis 1992;3:451–60.
5. Letai A, Kuter DJ. Cancer, coagulation, and anticoagulation. Oncologist 1999;4(6):443–9.
6. Rickles FR, Edwards RL. Activation of blood coagulation in cancer: Trousseau's syndrome revisited. Blood 1983;62(1):14–31.
7. Harrington KJ, Bateman AR, Syrigos KN, et al. Cancer-related thromboembolic disease in patients with solid tumours: a retrospective analysis. Ann Oncol 1997;8(7):669–73.
8. Pritchard KI, Paterson AH, Paul NA, et al. Increased thromboembolic complications with current tamoxifen and chemotherapy in a randomized trial of adjuvant therapy for women with breast cancer. National Cancer Institute of Canada Clinical trials Group Breast Cancer Site Group. J Clin Oncol 1996;14:2731–7.
9. Levine M, Gent M, Hirsh J, et al. The thrombogenic effect of anticancer drug therapy in women with stage II breast cancer. N Engl J Med 1988;318:404–7.
10. Holm T, Singnomklao T, Rutqvist LE, et al. Adjuvant preoperative radiotherapy in patients with rectal carcinoma. Adverse effects during long term follow-up of two randomized trials. Cancer (Phila) 1996;78(5):968–76.
11. Clagett GP, Anderson FA, Heith J, et al. Prevention of venous thromboembolism. Chest 1995;108:312–24.
12. Clagett PG, Reisch JS. Prevention of venous thromboembolism in general surgical patients. Result of a meta-analysis. Ann Surg 1988;208:227–40.
13. International Multicentre Trial. Prevention of fatal postoperative pulmonary embolism by low doses of heparin. Lancet 1975;11:45–51.
14. Bergqvist D, Burmark US, Flordal PA, et al. Low molecular weight heparin started before surgery as prophylaxis against deep vein thrombosis: 2500 versus 5000 XaI units in 2070 patients. Br J Surg 1995;82:496–501.

15. Agnelli G, Piovella F, Buoncristiani P, et al. Enoxaparin plus compression stocking compared with compression stockings alone in the prevention of venous thromboembolism after elective neurosurgery. N Engl J Med 1998;339(2):80–5.
16. Di Carlo V, Agnelli G, Prandoni P, et al. Dermatan sulphate for the prevention of postoperative venous thromboembolism in patients with cancer. DOS (Dermatan Sulphate in Oncologic Surgery) Study Group. Thromb Haemostasis 1999;82(1):30–4.
17. Bergqvist D, et al. Duration of prophylaxis against venous thromboembolism with enoxaparin after surgery for cancer. N Engl J Med 2002;346(13):975–80.
18. Levine M, Hirsh J, Gent M, et al. Double-blind randomised trial of a very-low-dose warfarin for prevention of thromboembolism in stage IV breast cancer. Lancet 1994;343(8902):886–9.
19. Bern MM, Lokich JJ, Wallach SR Jr, et al. Very low doses of warfarin can prevent thrombosis in central venous catheters. Ann Intern Med 1990;112:423–8.
20. Monreal M, Alastrue A, Rull M, et al. Upper extremity deep venous thrombosis in cancer patients with venous access devices: prophylaxis with a low molecular weight heparin (Fragmin). Thromb Haemostasis 1996;75(2):251–3.
21. Green D, Hull RD, Brant R, et al. Lower mortality in cancer patients treated with low molecular weight versus standard heparin [letter]. Lancet 1992;339:1476.
22. Siragusa S, Cosmi B, Piovella R, et al. Low molecular weight heparins and unfractionated heparin in the treatment of patients with acute venous thromboembolism: results of a meta-analysis. Am J Med 1996;100:269–77.
23. Kakkar AK, Levine MN, Kadzioal Z, et al. Low molecular weight heparin (LMWH) therapy and survival in advanced cancer. J Clin Oncol 2004;22(10):1944–8.
24. Klerk CP, Otten JMMB, et al. Malignancy and low molecular weight heparin therapy: the MALT trial. J Thromb Haemostasis 2003;I(suppl 1):abstract OC195.
25. Altinbas HSC, Er O, Ozkan M, et al. Prospective randomised study of epirubicine cyclophosphamide and vincristine. Combination chemotherapy (CEV), low molecular weight heparin (LMWH) in small cell lung cancer (SCLC). Proc Am Soc Clin Oncol 2001;20:235.

Prophylaxis of Venous Thromboembolism

Graham F. Pineo and Russell D. Hull

Introduction

Deep-vein thrombosis most commonly arises in the deep veins of the calf muscles or, less commonly, in the proximal deep veins of the leg. Deep-vein thrombosis confined to the calf veins is associated with a low risk of clinically important pulmonary embolism [1–3]. However, without treatment, approximately 20% of calf-vein thrombi extend into the proximal venous system where they may pose a serious and potentially life-threatening risk [3–5]. Untreated proximal venous thrombosis is associated with a 10% risk of fatal pulmonary embolism and at least a 50% risk of nonfatal pulmonary embolism or recurrent venous thrombosis [1–3]. Furthermore, the post-phlebitic syndrome is associated with extensive proximal venous thrombosis and carries its own long-term morbidity.

It is now well established that clinically important pulmonary emboli arise from thrombi in the proximal deep veins of the legs [3, 6–9]. Other less common sources of pulmonary embolism include the deep pelvic veins, renal veins, the inferior vena cava, the right heart, and, occasionally, the axillary veins. The clinical significance of pulmonary embolism depends on the size of the embolus and the cardiorespiratory reserve of the patient.

Various risk factors predispose to development of venous thromboembolism (Table 1).

University of Calgary, 601 South Tower, Foothills Hospital, 1403-29 Street NW, Calgary, Alberta, Canada T2N2T9

TABLE 1. Factors predisposing to the development of venous thromboembolism

Clinical risk factors	Inherited or acquired abnormalities
Surgical and nonsurgical trauma	Factor V Leiden mutation
Previous venous thromboembolism	Prothrombin G20210A mutation
Immobilization	Protein C deficiency
Malignant disease	Protein S deficiency
Heart disease	Antithrombin III deficiency
Leg paralysis	Anticardiolipin antibody syndrome
Age (>40 years)	Heparin-induced thrombocytopenia
Obesity	
Estrogens	
Parturition	

Prevention of Venous Thromboembolism

There are two approaches to the prevention of fatal pulmonary embolism: (a) primary prophylaxis is carried out using either drugs or physical methods that are effective for preventing deep-vein thrombosis; and (b) secondary prevention involves the early detection and treatment of subclinical venous thrombosis by screening postoperative patients with objective tests that are sensitive for venous thrombosis. Primary prophylaxis is preferred in most clinical circumstances [10, 11].

Without prophylaxis, the frequency of fatal pulmonary embolism ranges from 0.1% to 0.8% in patients undergoing elective general surgery [12–14], 2% to 3% in patients undergoing elective hip replacement [15], and 4% to 7% in patients undergoing surgery for a fractured hip [16]. The need for prophylaxis after elective hip replacement has been questioned because of the low incidence of fatal pulmonary embolism in patients participating in clinical trials [17]. However, review of data from the National Confidential Enquiry into Peri-Operative Deaths (NCEPOD) indicates that pulmonary embolism continues to be the most common cause of death following total hip replacement surgery; 35% of patients who died had pulmonary embolism confirmed at autopsy [18]. Factors increasing the risk of postoperative venous thrombosis include advanced age, malignancy, previous venous thromboembolism, obesity, heart failure, or paralysis (Table 1).

The ideal prophylactic agents are described in Table 2. Prophylactic measures most commonly used are low-dose or adjusted-dose unfractionated heparin, low molecular weight heparin, oral anticoagulants [international normalized ratio (INR), 2.0–3.0], and intermittent pneumatic compression. Recently, the pentasaccharide fondaparinux (Arixtra) has been approved for

TABLE 2. Features of an ideal prophylactic method for venous thromboembolism

Effective compared with placebo or active approaches
Safe
Good compliance with patient, nurses, and physicians
Ease of administration
No need for laboratory monitoring
Cost-effective

use in patients undergoing surgery for total hip or total knee replacement or for hip fracture.

There has been recent concern regarding the use of regional anesthesia in the form of intraspinal or epidural anesthesia and/or analgesia and the use of prophylactic anticoagulants. Spinal hematomas have been reported with the use of intravenous or subcutaneous heparin and warfarin treatment, but most of these complications occurred in patients with complex clinical problems [19]. With the advent of low molecular weight heparin and the increased use of regional anesthesia, concern was raised regarding the potential risk of neuraxial damage due to bleeding when both procedures are used together. Surveys among anesthetists in Europe suggested that the likelihood of spinal hematoma in this setting was remote [20, 21]. However, experience in the United States with the use of neuraxial anesthesia and analgesia and the postoperative administration of low molecular weight heparin has resulted in a number of case reports of spinal hematoma, many of which caused permanent neurological damage [22]. Many of these occurred with continued epidural analgesia, many of the procedures were traumatic, and several patients were on nonsteroidal antiinflammatory drugs [22]. Other risk factors appear to be age over 75 and female gender. At this stage, the Food and Drug Administration (FDA) has recommended caution when neuraxial anesthesia is used in the presence of low molecular weight heparin prophylaxis. The American Association of Regional Anesthesia Committee has recently reviewed these issues, and new guidelines have been published [23].

For patients receiving preoperative low molecular weight heparin, spinal anesthetic should be delayed for 10 to 12h after the low molecular weight heparin dose. Neuraxial procedures should be avoided in patients administered a dose of low molecular weight heparin 2h preoperatively (e.g., general surgery patients). Patients who are started on low molecular weight heparin postoperatively may safely undergo single injection or continuous catheter techniques for neuraxial anesthesia. If the twice-daily dosing schedule is used, the first dose of low molecular weight heparin should be administered no earlier than 24h postoperatively. Indwelling catheters should be removed before initiation of low molecular weight heparin, and the first dose should be given at least 2h after catheter removal. For patients on a once-daily regimen of low molecular weight heparin, the first postoperative dose should be administered 6 to 8h postoperatively, with the second postoperative dose being given 24h after the first dose. If indwelling neuraxial catheters are being used, the catheters should be removed a minimum of 10 to 12h after the last dose of low molecular weight heparin, with the subsequent dose to be given a minimum of 2h after catheter removal.

With the use of low-dose unfractionated heparin, there is no contraindication to the use of neuraxial techniques, but the risk of bleeding can be reduced by delay of the heparin until after the spinal tap, providing it is atraumatic. For patients receiving an initial dose of warfarin before surgery, the INR should be checked before neuraxial block. If neuraxial catheters are being used, the INR should be checked daily and the catheter should be removed when the INR is less than 1.5. It is recommended that fondaparinux be used with extreme caution because of its sustained antithrombotic effect, early postoperative dosing, and irreversibility of the antithrombotic effect.

Timing of Commencement of Prophylaxis

For patients undergoing general surgical procedures, the pattern of practice based on numerous clinical trials has been to start prophylaxis 2h preoperatively with either unfractionated heparin or low molecular weight heparin [24–29]. This approach has been shown to be both effective and safe, and indeed resulted in a significant decrease in the incidence of fatal pulmonary embolism in surgical patients [24, 25]. For patients undergoing high-risk orthopedic surgical procedures such as total hip or total knee replacement or surgery for hip fracture, because of concern about excess bleeding, commencement of prophylaxis has been delayed. Thus, in Europe, prophylaxis is commenced 10 to 12h preoperatively [30–37], whereas in North America, prophylaxis is usually started 12 to 24h postoperatively [38–45]. This difference in patterns of practice may account for the difference in the rates of postoperative venous thrombosis and bleeding in Europe and North America [46].

There is now good evidence that the timing of the initial administration of a prophylactic agent has a significant impact on the incidence of postoperative venous thrombosis. Starting low molecular weight heparin (dalteparin) at half the daily dose within 2h of hip replacement surgery followed by a further half dose 6 to 8h later and then using the usual once-daily dose significantly decreased the incidence of venous thrombosis when compared with placebo or warfarin [47, 48]. Compared with warfarin started the evening before surgery, the incidence of venographically proven deep-vein thrombosis was 25.8% versus 14.6% with low molecular weight heparin ($P = 0.006$). The incidence of proximal venous thrombosis was similar in the two groups. Although there was no difference in the incidence of major bleeding, patients on low molecular weight heparin had more bleeding complications involving the operative site, and a greater percentage of patients required postoperative transfusions [48].

In the North American Fragmin Trial, starting low molecular weight heparin (dalteparin) at half the usual daily dose within 2h before surgery or within 4 to 6h after surgery for total hip replacement significantly decreased the incidence of deep-vein thrombosis demonstrated by venography when compared with warfarin started the night of surgery [49]. The incidence of deep-vein thrombosis detected by venography was 10.7% for low molecular weight heparin started preoperatively, 13.1% for low molecular weight heparin started postoperatively, and 24% for patients on warfarin ($P < 0.001$). The incidence of proximal deep-vein thrombosis in the three groups was 0.8% for the two low molecular weight heparin groups versus 3.0% for the warfarin group ($P = 0.04$). There was no difference in the incidence of major bleeding reported by the principal investigators.

The results of the two studies comparing the early initiation of low molecular weight heparin with warfarin were compared with two previous studies where warfarin prophylaxis was compared with low molecular weight heparin started 12h preoperatively or 12 to 24h postoperatively [48, 49]. In a systematic review, it was shown that the incidence of postoperative venous thrombosis was significantly lower in the two clinical trials starting prophylaxis in close proximity to surgery compared with the studies where low molecular weight heparin was started either 12h preoperatively or 12 to 24h postoperatively (Figs. 1–3) [50]. There was no increase in the incidence of major bleeding.

Evidence from a number of other recent randomized clinical trials using newer antithrombotic agents started close to surgery suggests that the early commencement of prophylaxis plays a role in the improved efficacy of these agents when compared with accepted standards for prophylaxis. The antithrombin recombinant hirudin started 2h preoperatively was superior to the low molecular weight heparin (enoxaparin) started the night before surgery for both total and proximal deep-vein thrombosis [51]. Studies with the direct thrombin inhibitor melagatran (subcutaneous form) and ximelagatran (oral form) produced interesting results. When melagatran by subcutaneous injection twice daily was started immediately before surgery and continued for 2 to 3 days, followed by ximelagatran in different doses twice daily, the deep-vein thrombosis rates were either equivalent to or significantly lower than those seen with low molecular weight heparin (dalteparin) started the night before surgery in patients undergoing total hip or total knee

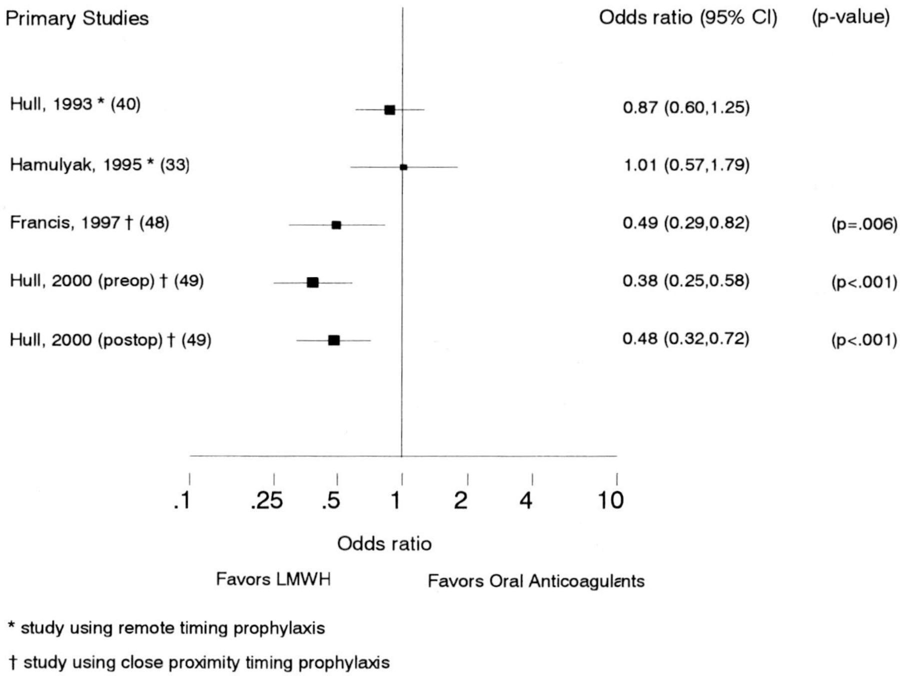

FIG. 1. Primary study odds ratios for all deep-vein thrombosis. Odds ratios are indicated by *boxes*. *Horizontal lines* represent 95% confidence intervals (CIs). Odds ratios less than 1.0 favor low molecular weight heparins (*LMWH*); odds ratios greater than 1.0 favor oral anticoagulants. (Adapted from Hull et al. [50] with permission)

replacement [52, 53]. When ximelagatran and low molecular weight heparin (enoxaparin) were started the morning after surgery, the venous thromboembolism rates were significantly lower with enoxaparin treatment, with no difference in major bleeding rates [54, 55].

Studies with the synthetic pentasaccharide fondaparinux (Arixtra) suggest that the timing of commencement of this agent may in part account for the superior efficacy when compared with low molecular weight heparin (enoxaparin). In a dose-finding study, fondaparinux was started 6h following surgery in five different doses and compared with enoxaparin started 12 to 24h after the end of surgery. Depending on the dose of fondaparinux, the deep-vein thrombosis rates were either equivalent to or significantly lower than those with enoxaparin [56]. In four phase 3 clinical trials, fondaparinux was started 6h following the end of surgery and given once daily, and compared with enoxaparin started either the night before surgery or 12 to 24h after the finish of surgery in patients undergoing total hip or total knee replacement or surgery for hip fracture [57–61]. These studies all showed

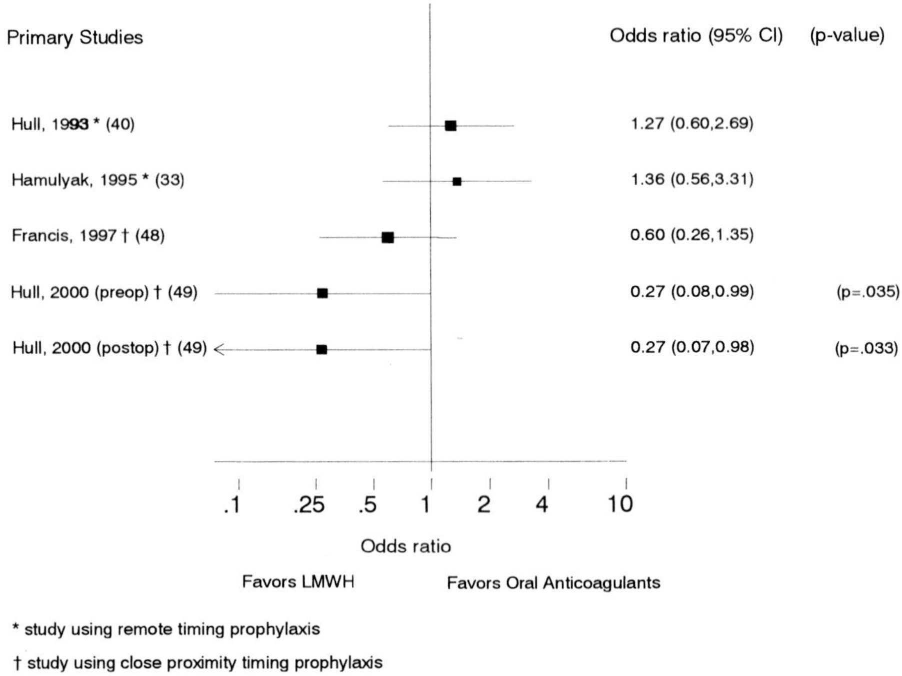

FIG. 2. Primary study odds ratios for proximal deep-vein thrombosis. Odds ratios are indicated by *boxes*. *Horizontal lines* represent 95% CIs. Odds ratios less than 1.0 favor low-molecular-weight heparins (*LMWH*); odds ratios greater than 1.0 favor oral anticoagulants. (Adapted from Hull et al. [50] with permission)

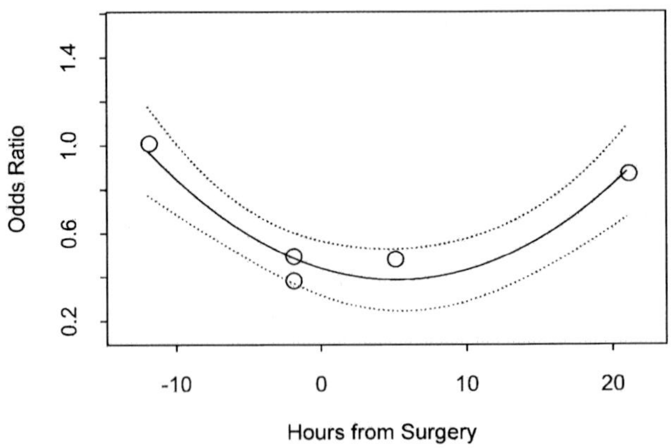

FIG. 3. Quadratic fit for study odds ratio for deep-vein thrombosis versus the number of hours from surgery for the first dose of low-molecular-weight heparin. The *upper and lower dashed lines* indicate the 95% CIs for the true odds ratio. (Adapted from Hull et al. [50] with permission)

fondaparinux to be superior to enoxaparin for the reduction of deep-vein thrombosis, although the decrease in the North American hip replacement study was not statistically significant. Other clinical trials, most of which are currently ongoing, have used a similar approach with the new agents starting 6 to 8 h postoperatively and compared with low molecular weight heparin started 12 to 24 h postoperatively.

Extended Out-of-Hospital Prophylaxis

It is widely recognized that the risk of developing deep-vein thrombosis increases after total hip arthroplasty [62]. The need for in-hospital prophylaxis has been firmly established. The Sixth ACCP Consensus Conference recommends anticoagulant prophylaxis for at least 7 to 10 days following elective total hip replacement surgery [28]. Although thromboprophylaxis is routinely administered for total hip replacement patients, it is commonly stopped at the time of discharge from hospital. In a recent epidemiological study by White and colleagues [63], a large linked hospital discharge database revealed the mean length of hospital stay after primary and revision total hip arthroplasty was 6.9 and 8.0 days, respectively. The period of risk for the development of venous thromboembolism was shown to extend well beyond this initial hospital stay [63]. In this study of hip arthroplasty patients, White et al. reported that 76% of thromboembolic cases were diagnosed after hospital discharge. The median time for diagnosing these thromboembolic events was 17 days after hip arthroplasty. The median time for diagnosing venous thromboembolism following total knee arthroplasty was 7 days, suggesting that extended prophylaxis may not be required in such knee patients.

There have been six randomized clinical trials comparing extended prophylaxis with low molecular weight heparin to placebo in patients undergoing total hip replacement who have received either low molecular weight heparin (enoxaparin or dalteparin) or warfarin for in-hospital prophylaxis [34–37, 44, 64]. All these trials indicated that deep-vein thrombosis rates were decreased with extended prophylaxis. A systematic review of all six clinical trials demonstrated a significant decrease in both total and proximal deep-vein thrombosis as demonstrated by bilateral venography, but also demonstrated a significant decrease in symptomatic venous thromboembolism occurring during the treatment period [65]. There was no major bleeding in the out-of-hospital phase of any of these trials, indicating that the risk-to-benefit ratio strongly favored extended prophylaxis (Figs. 4–6).

Extended prophylaxis with acecoumarol was compared with low molecular weight heparin for extended prophylaxis up to 30 days following total hip replacement. Deep-vein thrombosis rates were similar, but there was signifi-

Study	Year	Expt n/N (%)	Ctrl n/N (%)	Relative Risk (95% CI Fixed)	Weight (%)	Relative Risk (95% CI Fixed)	p Value
Bergqvist (34)	1996	21/117 (17.9)	45/116 (38.8)		28.6	0.46 (0.30, 0.73)	0.001
Planes (35)	1996	6/85 (7.1)	17/88 (19.3)		10.6	0.37 (0.15, 0.88)	0.025
Dahl (36)	1997	11/93 (11.8)	23/89 (25.8)		14.9	0.46 (0.24, 0.88)	0.020
Lassen (37)	1998	5/113 (4.4)	12/102 (11.8)		8.0	0.38 (0.14, 1.03)	0.057
Hull (64)	2000	14/291 (4.8)	14/133 (10.5)		12.2	0.46 (0.22, 0.93)	0.031
Comp (44)	2001	15/152 (9.9)	39/138 (28.2)		25.9	0.35 (0.20, 0.60)	<0.001
Total		72/911 (7.9)	150/666 (22.5)		100.0	0.41 (0.32, 0.54)	<0.001

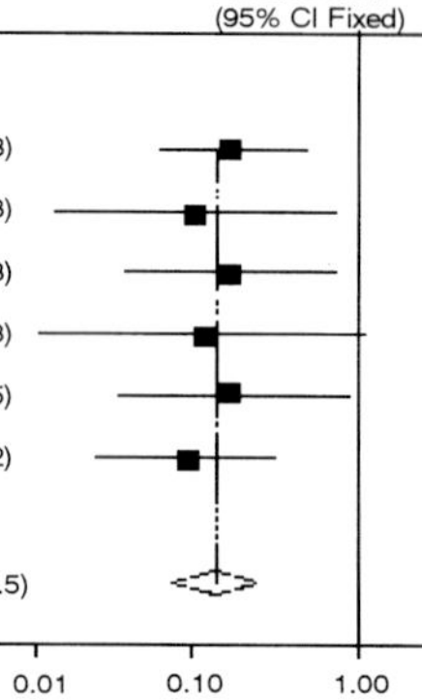

FIG. 4. The relative risk for all deep-vein thrombosis during the out-of-hospital time interval; summary and individual study results. (Adapted from Hull et al. [65] with permission)

Study	Year	Expt n/N (%)	Ctrl n/N (%)	Relative Risk (95% CI Fixed)	Weight (%)	Relative Risk (95% CI Fixed)	p Value
Bergqvist (34)	1996	8/117 (6.8)	28/116 (24.1)		35.2	0.28 (0.13, 0.60)	0.001
Planes (35)	1996	5/85 (5.9)	7/88 (8.0)		8.6	0.74 (0.24, 2.24)	0.594
Dahl (36)	1997	4/93 (4.3)	9/89 (10.1)		11.5	0.43 (0.14, 1.33)	0.142
Lassen (37)	1998	1/111 (0.9)	5/101 (5.0)		6.6	0.18 (0.02, 1.53)	0.117
Hull (64)	2000	3/308 (1.0)	7/146 (4.8)		11.9	0.20 (0.05, 0.77)	0.020
Comp (44)	2001	5/152 (3.3)	20/138 (14.5)		26.2	0.23 (0.19, 0.59)	0.002
Total		26/866 (3.0)	76/678 (11.2)		100.0	0.31 (0.20, 0.47)	<0.001

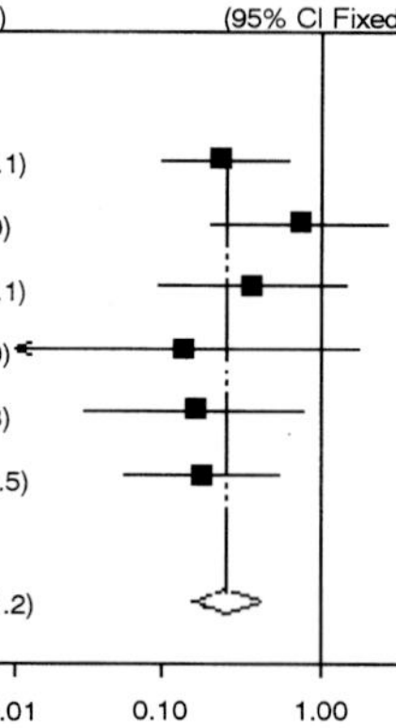

FIG. 5. The relative risk for proximal deep-vein thrombosis during the out-of-hospital time interval: summary and individual study results. (Adapted from Hull et al. [65] with permission)

cantly more bleeding with acecoumarol [66]. Also, extended prophylaxis with warfarin up to 4 weeks was superior to warfarin continued for 1 week in patients undergoing total hip replacement surgery [67]. In the PENTHIFRA-plus Study, continuation of fondaparinux for 4 weeks was compared with 7 days of fondaparinux followed by placebo [68]. There was a significant decrease in both venographic evidence of recurrent deep-vein thrombosis

Study	Year	Expt n/N (%)	Ctrl n/N (%)	Relative Risk (95% CI Fixed)	Weight (%)	Relative Risk (95% CI Fixed)	p Value
Bergqvist (34)	1996	2/131 (1.5)	10/131 (7.6)		26.3	0.20 (0.04, 0.90)	0.035
Planes (35)	1996	3/90 (3.3)	7/89 (7.9)		18.5	0.42 (0.11, 1.59)	0.203
Dahl (36)	1997	4/117 (3.4)	6/110 (5.5)		16.3	0.63 (0.18, 2.16)	0.460
Lassen (37)	1998	2/140 (1.4)	3/141 (2.1)		7.9	0.67 (0.11, 3.96)	0.660
Hull (64)	2000	4/389 (1.0)	3/180 (1.7)		10.8	0.62 (0.14, 2.73)	0.524
Comp (44)	2001	0/224 (0.0)	7/211 (3.3)		20.3	0.06 (0.00, 1.09)	0.058
Total		15/1091 (1.4)	36/862 (4.2)		100.0	0.36 (0.20, 0.67)	<0.001

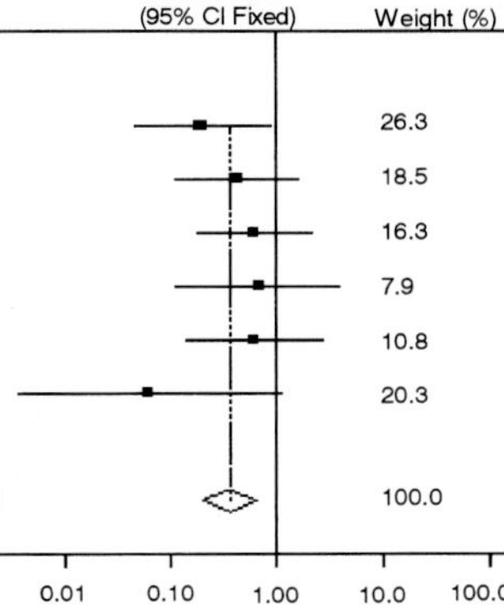

FIG. 6. The relative risk for symptomatic venous thromboembolism during the out-of-hospital time interval: summary and individual study results. (Adapted from Hull et al. [65] with permission)

and symptomatic venous thromboembolism with the extended use of fondaparinux. Extended prophylaxis to day 28 in patients undergoing total knee replacement did not significantly lower the rates of venous thrombosis when compared with 7 to 10 days of prophylaxis with low molecular weight heparin [44].

In patients undergoing cancer surgery, extended prophylaxis up to 25 to 31 days with low molecular weight heparin was superior to prophylaxis for 6 to 10 days [69]. Extended prophylaxis is currently being studied in high-risk medical patients. The advent of effective oral agents will simplify the approach to extended prophylaxis, but concerns about cost will remain a problem.

Specific Prophylactic Measures

Patterns of clinical practice with respect to the prevention of venous thromboembolism and the appropriate use of anticoagulants for the treatment of thrombotic disease have been influenced very strongly by recent consensus conferences [28, 70]. Recommendations from the Sixth American College of Chest Physicians Consensus Conference on Antithrombotic Therapy [28] and the International Consensus Statement on the Prevention of Venous Thromboembolism [70] have recently been published. Rules of evidence for assessing the literature were applied to all recommendations regarding prevention and treatment of venous thrombosis, thereby indicating which recommendations were based on rigorous randomized trials, which were based on extrapolation of evidence from related clinical disorders, and which were based only on nonrandomized clinical trials or case series [28].

Low Molecular Weight Heparin

A number of low molecular weight heparins have been evaluated by randomized clinical trials in moderate-risk general surgical patients including many who underwent cancer surgery [26, 27, 29, 71–73]. In randomized clinical trials comparing low molecular weight heparin with unfractionated heparin, the low molecular weight heparins given once or twice daily have been shown to be as effective or more effective in preventing thrombosis [26, 27, 29, 71–73]. In most of the trials, similarly low frequencies of bleeding for low molecular weight heparin and low-dose unfractionated heparin were documented [26, 27].

A number of randomized control trials have been performed with low molecular weight heparin, comparing it with either unfractionated heparin or warfarin for the prevention of venous thrombosis following total hip replacement. The most recent trials using bilateral venography are shown in Table 3 [30–40, 44, 49]. The drugs under investigation and their dosage schedules vary from one clinical trial to another, making comparisons across trials difficult. Furthermore, it has been shown that even within the same clinical trial there can be considerable intercenter variability [40]. Major bleeding rates and definitions of major bleeding vary across trials as well, making comparisons difficult.

Although the number of patients undergoing total knee replacement now equals those undergoing total hip replacements, there have been fewer trials in this patient population. Recent clinical trials comparing low molecular weight heparin with warfarin are shown in Table 4 [33, 40, 42, 43]. Although the rates of deep-vein thrombosis with low molecular weight heparin are significantly lower than those with warfarin, the rates continue to be high.

Multiple meta-analyses have shown that low molecular weight heparin and low-dose heparin are equally effective in preventing venous thrombosis in general surgery [74–76], but low molecular weight heparin is more effective in orthopedic surgery [74–79]. Bleeding rates were higher with low-dose heparin in patients undergoing general surgery.

In medical patients, earlier studies showed that both low-dose heparin and low molecular weight heparin were superior to placebo in preventing venous thrombosis in high-risk medical patients. Meta-analysis of the early trials indicated equal efficacy for low-dose heparin and low molecular weight heparin in the prevention of venous thromboembolism, but there was more bleeding with low-dose heparin [78]. More recently, in large multicenter

TABLE 3. Recent randomized trials of low molecular weight heparin versus heparin or warfarin prophylaxis for deep-vein thrombosis following hip replacement surgery: total deep-vein thrombosis and major bleeding

Reference	Treatment	No. of patients	Total deep-vein thrombosis (%)	Major bleeding (%)
Levine et al. [38]	Enoxaparin	258	19.4	3.3
	Unfractionated heparin	263	23.3	5.7
Leyvraz et al. [30]	Nadroparin	198	12.6	0.5
	Unfractionated heparin	199	16.0	1.5
Eriksson et al. [31]	Dalteparin	67	30.2	1.4[a]
	Unfractionated heparin	68	42.4	7.4
Planes et al. [32]	Enoxaparin	120	12.5	1.6
	Heparin	108	25.0	0
Colwell et al. [39]	Enoxaparin	136	21.0	4.0
	Enoxaparin	136	6.0	1.0
	Heparin	142	1.5	6.0
Hull et al. [40]	Tinzaparin	332	21.0	2.8
	Warfarin	340	23.0	1.5
Hamulyak et al. [33]	Nadroparin	195	13.8	1.5[b]
	Warfarin	196	13.8	2.3
Francis et al. [48]	Dalteparin	192	15.0	2.0
	Warfarin	190	26.0	1.0
Hull et al. [49]	Dalteparin	496	10.7	2.8
	Dalteparin	487	13.1	1.8
	Warfarin	489	24.0	2.0

[a] Serious bleeding
[b] Clinically important plus minor bleeding for combined hip and knee replacement patients

TABLE 4. Randomized control trials of low molecular weight heparin prophylaxis versus warfarin for deep-vein thrombosis following total knee replacement: total deep-vein thrombosis and major bleeding

Reference	Treatment	No. of patients	Total deep-vein thrombosis (%)	Major bleeding (%)
Hull et al. [40]	Tinzaparin	317	45.0	0.9
	Warfarin	324	54.0	2.0
Leclerc et al. [42]	Enoxaparin	206	37.0	2.1
	Warfarin	211	52.0	1.8
Heit et al. [43]	Ardeparin	232	27.0[a]	7.9[b]
	Warfarin	222	38.0	4.4
Hamulyak et al. [33]	Nadroparin	65	24.6	1.5[c]
	Warfarin	61	37.7	2.3

[a] Venogram on operated leg only
[b] Overt bleeding, total
[c] Clinically important and minor bleeding for combined hip and knee replacement patients

clinical trials, low molecular weight heparin was shown to significantly reduce the incidence of venous thromboembolism in high-risk medical patients when compared with placebo [79–81]. In the MEDENOX Study, enoxaparin 40 mg was found to be superior to enoxaparin 20 mg or placebo in the reduction of venographically demonstrated deep-vein thrombosis [79]. In the PREVENT Study, dalteparin 5000 units was superior to placebo in the prevention of symptomatic venous thromboembolism plus proximal deep-vein thrombosis seen on screening ultrasound at day 21 in the prevention of venous thromboembolism [80]. Low molecular weight heparin (enoxaparin) and low-dose heparin showed comparable results following ischemic stroke in terms of efficacy and safety [81]. Low molecular weight heparin was superior to low-dose heparin in preventing venous thromboembolism in patients suffering multiple trauma [82].

Low-Dose Heparin

The effectiveness of low-dose unfractionated heparin for preventing deep-vein thrombosis following general surgery has been established by multiple randomized clinical trials [24–27]. Low-dose subcutaneous heparin is usually given in a dose of 5000 units 2 h preoperatively and every 8 or 12 h postoperatively. Most of the patients in these trials underwent abdominothoracic surgery, particularly for gastrointestinal disease, but patients having gynecological and urological surgery as well as mastectomies or vascular procedures were also included. Pooled data from meta-analyses confirm that low-dose heparin significantly reduces the incidence of all deep-vein thrombosis, proximal deep-vein thrombosis, and all pulmonary emboli including fatal pulmonary emboli [24, 74–77]. The International Multicentre Trial also established the effectiveness of low-dose heparin for preventing fatal pulmonary embolism, a clinically and significantly striking reduction from 0.7% to 0.1% ($P < 0.005$) [23].

The incidence of major bleeding complications is not increased by low-dose heparin, but there is an increase in minor wound hematomas. The platelet count should be monitored regularly in all patients on low-dose heparin to detect the rare but significant development of heparin-induced thrombocytopenia.

Intermittent Leg Compression

The use of intermittent pneumatic leg compression prevents venous thrombosis by enhancing blood flow in the deep veins of the legs, thereby preventing venous stasis. It also increases blood fibrinolytic activity, which may contribute to its antithrombotic properties. Intermittent pneumatic leg compression is effective for preventing venous thrombosis following cardiac surgery [89] and in patients undergoing neurosurgery [83–85]. In patients undergoing hip surgery, intermittent pneumatic compression of the calf is effective for preventing calf vein thrombosis, but it is less effective against proximal vein thrombosis than warfarin sodium [86, 87]. Intermittent pneumatic compression of the calf decreased venous thrombosis following knee replacement [88, 89].

With a shortened hospital stay, use of intermittent pneumatic compression becomes of limited value. A greater problem, however, is one of compliance [90, 91]. In addition to poor compliance, a recent study documented the fact that key outcome-related parameters such as the rate of pressure rise and the maximum pressure applied to various parts of the leg were less than anticipated most of the time in patients having intermittent pneumatic compression following elective hip surgery [91]. Disappointingly, an intensive nursing training program did not improve these outcomes.

Graduated Compression Stockings

Graduated compression stockings are a simple, safe, and moderately effective form of thromboprophylaxis. It is by no means clear how graduated compression stockings achieve a thromboprophylactic effect. It has been shown that they increase the velocity of venous blood flow, and thus graduated compression stockings are recommended in low-risk patients and as an adjunct in those with medium and high risk [92–94]. The only major contraindication is peripheral vascular disease. The majority of studies in patients undergoing general abdominal and gynecological procedures have shown a reduction in the incidence of deep-vein thrombosis. A comprehensive meta-analysis concluded that, in studies using objective methods, there was a highly significant risk reduction of 68% in patients at moderate risk of postoperative thromboembolism [94]. However, there is no conclusive evidence that graduated compression stockings are effective in reducing the incidence of fatal and nonfatal pulmonary embolism. It is not known whether wearing graduated compression stockings following discharge from hospital is efficacious.

Oral Anticoagulants

For prophylaxis, oral anticoagulants (coumarin derivatives) can be commenced preoperatively, at the time of surgery, or in the early postoperative period [95]. Oral anticoagulants commenced at the time of surgery or in the early postoperative period may not prevent small venous thrombi from forming during surgery, or soon after surgery, because the antithrombotic effect is not achieved until the third or fourth postoperative day. However, oral anticoagulants are effective in inhibiting the extension of these thrombi, thereby preventing clinically important venous thromboembolism.

The postoperative use of warfarin following total hip or total knee replacement surgery has been compared with low molecular weight heparin [33, 40, 48, 49, 96, 97] or intermittent pneumatic compression [87, 97], with little or no difference in the incidence of postoperative venous thrombosis or bleeding. However, more recent studies using earlier intervention with low molecular weight heparin have demonstrated superior efficacy when compared with warfarin, closely controlled using a warfarin nomogram [49]. Another clinical trial using clinical endpoints for venous thromboembolism demonstrated superior efficacy of low molecular weight heparin, although the majority of patients on warfarin had an INR of less than 2 [96].

In patients with hip fractures, warfarin was more effective than either aspirin or placebo [98]. Compared with placebo, very low doses of oral anticoagulants (warfarin 1 mg per day) decreased the postoperative thrombosis rate in patients undergoing gynecological surgery or major general surgery [99].

New Antithrombotic Agents

The pentasaccharide fondaparinux is a highly selective Factor X inhibitor with a high affinity for antithrombin. When fondaparinux binds to antithrombin, it induces a confirmational change which markedly increases the rate of Factor Xa inhibition. When antithrombin then binds to activated Factor X, the fondaparinux is released and thus continues the process. Inhibition of Xa leads to less generation of thrombin, but unlike other antithrombotic agents, fondaparinux does not inhibit other coagulation proteins or affect platelet function or aggregation. Fondaparinux has a long half-life (17 h), permitting once-daily dosing. Fondaparinux has the further advantage of being a wholly synthetic molecule, which is not dependant on animal sources as are the heparins, and it does not produce heparin-associated antibodies. Of some concern is the fact that the antithrombotic activity cannot be blocked by any of the known agents, and the FDA has mandated that caution be used in elderly patients who may have decreased renal function because of a concern that there may be accumulation of the drug. It was also stated "differences in efficacy and safety between Arixtra and the comparator may have been influenced by factors such as the timing of the first dose of the drug after surgery," an observation that had previously been made [100].

In a dose-finding study, fondaparinux was shown to have a highly reproducible and linear dose-dependent inhibition of thrombosis, as well as a dose-dependent increase in major bleeding [56]. Fondaparinux has been compared with the low molecular weight heparin enoxaparin in more than 7000 patients undergoing orthopedic procedures in phase 3 clinical trials [57–60]. The fondaparinux protocol was the same in all four studies (i.e., 2.5 mg s.c. started 6 h after the operation with the second injection 12 h or longer after the first). In the hip fracture study, enoxaparin 40 mg was started an average of 18 h postoperatively, in the knee replacement study enoxaparin 30 mg twice daily an average of 21 h postoperatively, in the European hip replacement study enoxaparin 40 mg was started 12 h preoperatively, and in the North American hip replacement study enoxaparin 30 mg twice daily was started a mean of 13 h postoperatively. In the hip fracture study, there was a significant decrease in both total and proximal deep-vein thrombosis rates with fondaparinux with no difference in the major bleeding rates, although minor bleeding was increased with fondaparinux. Extended use of fondaparinux resulted in a significant decrease in the incidence of venous thrombosis compared to placebo [67]. In the knee replacement study, there was a significant decrease in the total deep-vein thrombosis rates with fondaparinux but proximal rates were similar; however, there was a significant increase in major bleeding as indicated by the bleeding index in the fondaparinux group [58]. In the European total hip replacement study, there was a significant decrease in both total and proximal deep-vein thrombosis rates in the fondaparinux group [59], whereas in the North American study there was a significant difference in venographically proven distal deep-vein thrombosis but not for proximal deep-vein thrombosis [60]. In both studies the bleeding index was similar in both groups. When all studies were pooled there was a significant decrease in both total and proximal deep-vein thrombosis rates with fondaparinux but no difference in the incidence of symptomatic events [61]. The incidence of major bleeding was increased in the fondaparinux group [61].

The specific direct thrombin inhibitor melagatran (subcutaneous form) or ximelagatran (oral form) has undergone extensive study. In the first study, subcutaneous melagatran in three doses was given twice daily for 2 days beginning immediately before surgery with the second dose being on the evening of surgery, and on day 3 oral ximelagatran in three different doses was started in a twice-daily fashion for 6 to 9 days [52]. The control was dalteparin 5000 units started the evening before total hip or knee replacement surgery and continued daily. Bilateral venography showed there was no difference in total or proximal deep-vein thrombosis rates within the various groups. In the second study (METHRO II), a combination of subcutaneous melagatran starting immediately before surgery and continued twice daily for 2 to 3 days in four dose levels was followed by ximelagatran in four different doses orally twice daily and compared with dalteparin 5000 units started the evening before total hip or knee replacement surgery [53]. A highly significant dose-dependent decrease in deep-vein thrombosis rates was seen for both total hip and total knee replacement patients. Also, a dose-dependent decrease in proximal deep-vein thrombosis and pulmonary embolism was found in the total population. Total bleeding was not significantly different between the treatment groups.

In METHRO-III, melagatran was initiated 4 to 12h postoperatively and given twice daily for 3 days followed by oral ximelagatran and compared with the enoxaparin started 12h preoperatively [54]. There was a significant increase in total venous thromboembolism with the melagatran-ximelagatran in patients undergoing total hip replacement surgery but comparable rates for those having total knee replacement surgery. The incidence of proximal deep-vein thrombosis, pulmonary embolism, and bleeding was comparable in the two groups.

In the EXPRESS Study, the preoperative study dose of melagatran was re-introduced at 2mg, and subsequent twice-daily doses were 3mg for 1 to 3 days followed by oral ximelagatran [101]. In the total hip and total knee replacement surgery patients there was a significant decrease in the incidence of proximal deep-vein thrombosis and/or pulmonary embolism as well as total venous thromboembolism with use of the melagatran-ximelagatran. Excessive bleeding as judged by the investigator was higher in the melagatran-ximelagatran group.

Studies in North America have used only the oral ximelagatran started postoperatively. In a dose-finding study in patients undergoing total knee replacement surgery, the highest dose of ximelagatran used (24mg twice daily) was as effective as enoxaparin 30mg twice daily subcutaneously, both started 12 to 24h postoperatively.

In a phase II study in patients undergoing total hip replacement surgery, ximelagatran 24mg twice daily was compared with enoxaparin 30mg twice daily, both initiated the morning after surgery [54]. Enoxaparin-treated patients had significantly fewer events of venous thromboembolism (venographic and symptomatic venous thromboembolism) compared with ximelagatran-treated patients. Bleeding rates were low and comparable between the groups.

In a phase III study in patients undergoing total knee replacement surgery, ximelagatran 24mg bid started postoperatively was compared with warfarin begun on the evening of surgery with a target INR of 1.8 to 3.0 [55]. The incidence of deep-vein thrombosis demonstrated on unilateral venography was comparable. There was no difference in the incidence of bleeding. In the EXALT A Study, patients undergoing total knee replacement surgery received either ximelagatran 36mg twice daily or 24mg twice daily and compared with warfarin as before [102]. The composite endpoint of deep-vein thrombosis, confirmed symptomatic deep-vein thrombosis or pulmonary embolism, or death was lower in the ximelagatran 36 mg twice-daily group, although there were no statistically significant differences between the groups for proximal deep-vein thrombosis, pulmonary embolism, or death. Also there was no difference in the incidence of major bleeding, blood loss, or transfusion volumes. In a larger study (EXALT B), ximelagatran 36 mg twice daily is being compared to warfarin in patients undergoing total knee replacement.

Specific Recommendations

High-Risk Patients

- Elective hip replacement:
  - HInitial prophylaxis: low molecular weight heparin, fondaparinux, warfarin
  - Extended prophylaxis: low molecular weight heparin, warfarin
- Elective knee replacement:
  - Low molecular weight heparin, initial fondaparinux, warfarin
- Hip fracture:
  - Initial prophylaxis: fondaparinux, low molecular weight heparin, and warfarin
  - Extended prophylaxis: fondaparinux
- Multiple trauma:
  - Low molecular weight heparin with or without intermittent pneumatic compression
- Acute spinal cord injury with paralysis:
  - Initial intermittent pneumatic compression followed by low molecular weight heparin

Moderate-Risk Patients

- Neurosurgery:
  - Intermittent pneumatic compression followed by low molecular weight heparin or low-dose heparin
- General abdominal thoracic or gynecological surgery:
  - Low-dose heparin, low molecular weight heparin
- Cancer surgery:
  - Low molecular weight heparin or low-dose heparin
  - Extended prophylaxis: low molecular weight heparin

Low-Risk Patients

- Early ambulation with or without graduated compression stockings

Medical Patients

- Moderate- to high-risk patients (congestive heart failure, acute respiratory failure, sepsis, and other patients temporarily immobilized):
  - Low molecular weight heparin, low-dose heparin

Conclusions

There are now effective measures for the prevention of venous thromboembolism in most medical and surgical conditions. Based on information from level 1 clinical trials and systematic reviews, recommendations for the prevention of venous thromboembolism can be made for most circumstances encountered by the physician or surgeon. Where such information is not available, recommendations must be based on extrapolation from similar circumstances in which the risk reduction is known. Unfortunately, even when effective prophylactic agents are available they are commonly not applied, particularly in medical patients at risk of venous thromboembolism. Pulmonary embolism is one of the most preventable causes of death in hospital practice. The ultimate goal of prophylaxis should be the elimination of fatal pulmonary embolism in medical and surgical patients, a goal that at the present time is still unfulfilled.

References

1. Hull RD, Hirsh J, Carter CJ, et al. Diagnostic efficacy of impedance plethysmography for clinically suspected deep vein thrombosis: a randomized trial. Ann Intern Med 1985;102:21–8.
2. Huisman MV, Buller HR, ten Cate JW, et al. Serial impedance plethysmography for suspected deep venous thrombosis in outpatients. The Amsterdam General Practitioner Study. N Engl J Med 1986;314:823–8.
3. Kakkar VV, Howe CT, Flanc C, et al. Natural history of postoperative deep vein thrombosis. Lancet 1969;2:230–3.
4. Lagerstedt CI, Olsson CG, Fagher BO, et al. Need for long term anticoagulant treatment in symptomatic calf vein thrombosis. Lancet 1985;2:515–18.
5. Lohr JM, James KV, Deshmukh RM, et al. Calf vein thrombi are not a benign finding. Am J Surg 1995;170:86–90.
6. Moser KM, Le Moine JR. Is embolic risk conditioned by location of deep venous thrombosis? Ann Intern Med 1981;94:439–44.
7. Sevitt S, Gallagher N. Venous thrombosis and pulmonary embolism. A clinicopathological study in injured and burned patients. Br J Surg 1961;48:475–89.
8. Mavor GE, Galloway JMD. The iliofemoral venous segment as a source of pulmonary emboli. Lancet 1967;1:871–4.
9. Hull RD, Hirsh J, Carter CJ, et al. Diagnostic value of ventilation-perfusion lung scanning in patients with suspected pulmonary embolism. Chest 1985;88:819–28.

10. Salzman EW, Davies GC. Prophylaxis of venous thromboembolism. Analysis of cost-effectiveness. Ann Surg 1980;191:207–18.
11. Hull R, Hirsh J, Sackett DL, et al. Cost-effectiveness of primary and secondary prevention of fatal pulmonary embolism in high risk surgical patients. CMAJ 1982;127:990–5.
12. Kakkar VV, Adams PC. Preventive and therapeutic approach to thromboembolic disease and pulmonary embolism: can death from pulmonary embolism be prevented? J Am Coll Cardiol 1986;8(6 suppl B):146B–58B.
13. Skinner DB, Salzman EW. Anticoagulant prophylaxis in surgical patients. Surg Gynecol Obstet 1967;125:741–6.
14. Shephard RM Jr, White HA, Shirkey AL. Anticoagulant prophylaxis of thromboembolism in post-surgical patients. Am J Surg 1966;112:698–702.
15. Coventry MB, Nolan DR, Beckenbaugh RD. "Delayed" prophylactic anticoagulation: a study of results and complications in 2,012 total hip arthoplasties. J Bone Joint Surg [Am] 1973;55:1487–92.
16. Eskeland G, Solheim K, Skjorten F. Anticoagulant prophylaxis, thromboembolism and mortality in elderly patients with hip fracture: a controlled clinical trial. Acta Chir Scand 1966;131:16–29.
17. Murray DW, Britton AR, Bulstrode CJK. Thromboprophylaxis and death after total hip replacement. J Bone Joint Surg [Br] 1996;78(6):863–70.
18. Campling EA, Devlin HB, Hoile RW, et al. The report of the national confidential enquiry into perioperative deaths (NCEPOD) 1991/92. London HMS0.
19. Vandermeulen EP, Van Aken H, Vermylen J. Anticoagulants and spinal-epidural anesthesia. Anesth Analg 1994;79:1165–1177.
20. Bergqvist D, Lindblad B, Matzsch T. Risk of combining low molecular weight heparin for thromboprophylaxis and epidural or spinal anesthesia. Semin Thromb Hemost 1993;19(suppl 1):147–51.
21. Dahlgren N, Tornebrandt K. Neurological complications after anaesthesia; a follow-up of 18,000 spinal and epidural anaesthetics performed over three years. Acta Anaesthesiol Scand 1995;39:872–80.
22. Horlocker TT, Heit JA. Low molecular weight heparin: biochemistry, pharmacology, perioperative prophylaxis regimens, and guidelines for regional anesthetic management. Anesth Analg 1997;85:874–85.
23. Horlocker TT, Wedel DJ, Benzon H, et al. Regional anesthesia in the anticoagulated patient: defining the risks (the second ASRA Consensus Conference on Neuraxial Anesthesia and Anticoagulation). Reg Anesth Pain Med 2003;28(3):172–97.
24. International Multicentre Trial. Prevention of fatal postoperative pulmonary embolism by low doses of heparin. Lancet 1975;2:45–51.
25. Collins R, Scrimgeour A, Yusef S, et al. Reduction in fatal pulmonary embolism and venous thrombosis by perioperative administration of subcutaneous heparin. N Engl J Med 1988;318:1162–73.
26. Kakkar VV, Cohen AT, Edmonson RA. Low molecular weight versus standard heparin for prevention of venous thromboembolism after major abdominal surgery. Lancet 1993;341:259–65.
27. Kakkar VV, Boeckl O, Boneau B, et al. Efficacy and safety of a low molecular weight heparin and standard unfractionated heparin for prophylaxis of postoperative venous thromboembolism: European multicenter trial. World J Surg 1997;21:2–9.
28. Geerts WH, Heit JA, Clagett GP, et al. Prevention of venous thromboembolism. Chest (Suppl) 2001;119:132S–75S.

29. Bergqvist D, Burmark US, Flordal PA, et al. Low molecular weight heparin started before surgery as prophylaxis against deep vein thrombosis: 2500 versus 5000 Xal units in 2070 patients. Br J Surg 1995;82:496–501.
30. Leyvraz PF, Bachmann F, Hoek J, et al. Prevention of deep vein thrombosis after hip replacement: randomised comparison between unfractionated heparin and low molecular weight heparin. BMJ 1991;303:543–8.
31. Eriksson BI, Kälebo P, Anthymyr BA, et al. Prevention of deep vein thrombosis and pulmonary embolism after total hip replacement. J Bone Joint Surg [Am] 1991;73A(4):484–93.
32. Planes A, Vochelle N, Fagola M, et al. Prevention of deep vein thrombosis after total hip replacement: the effect of low molecular weight heparin with spinal and general anaesthesia. J Bone Joint Surg [Br] 1991;73:418–22.
33. Hamulyak, K, Lensing AW, van der Meer J, et al. Subcutaneous low-molecular-weight heparin or oral anticoagulants for the prevention of deep-vein thrombosis in elective hip and knee replacement? Thromb Haemostasis 1995;74(6):1428–31.
34. Bergqvist D, Benoni G, Bjorgell O, et al. Low molecular weight heparin (enoxaparin) as prophylaxis against venous thromboembolism after total hip replacement. N Engl J Med 1996;335(10):696–700.
35. Planes A, Vochelle N, Darmon JY, et al. Risk of deep-venous thrombosis after hospital discharge in patients having undergone total hip replacement: double-blind randomized comparison of enoxaparin versus placebo. Lancet 1996;348: 224–8.
36. Dahl OE, Andreassen G, Aspelin T, et al. Prolonged thromboprophylaxis following hip replacement surgery—results of a double-blind, prospective, randomized, placebo-controlled study with dalteparin (Fragmin). Thromb Haemostais 1997;77(1): 26–31.
37. Lassen MR, Borris LC, Anderson BS, et al. Efficacy and safety of prolonged thromboprophylaxis with a low-molecular-weight heparin (dalteparin) after total hip arthroplasty—the Danish prolonged prophylaxis (DaPP) study. Thromb Res 1998;89:281–7.
38. Levine MN, Hirsh J, Gent M, et al. Prevention of deep vein thrombosis after elective hip surgery: a randomized trial comparing low molecular weight heparin with standard unfractionated heparin. Ann Intern Med 1991;114(7):545–51.
39. Colwell CW Jr, Spiro TE, Trowbridge AA, et al. Use of enoxaparin, a low molecular weight heparin and unfractionated heparin for the prevention of deep venous thrombosis after elective hip replacement. J Bone Joint Surg [Am] 1994;76(1):3–14.
40. Hull RD, Raskob G, Pineo G, et al. A comparison of subcutaneous low-molecular-weight heparin with warfarin sodium for prophylaxis against deep-vein thrombosis after hip or knee implantation. N Engl J Med 1993;329(19):1370–6.
41. Leclerc JR, Geerts WH, Desjardins L, et al. Prevention of deep vein thrombosis after major knee surgery—a randomised, double-blind trial comparing a low molecular weight heparin fragment (enoxaparin) to placebo. Thromb Haemostasis 1992;67(4):417–23.
42. Leclerc JR, Geerts WH, Desjardins L, et al. Prevention of venous thromboembolism after knee arthroplasty—a randomized, double-blind trial comparing enoxaparin with warfarin. Ann Intern Med 1996;124:619–26.
43. Heit JA, Berkowitz SD, Bona R, et al. Efficacy and safety of low molecular weight heparin (ardeparin sodium) compared to warfarin for the prevention of venous thromboembolism after total knee replacement surgery: a double blind, dose ranging study. Thromb Haemostasis 1997;77(1):32–8.

44. Comp PC, Spiro TE, Friedman RJ, et al. Prolonged enoxaparin therapy to prevent venous thromboembolism after primary hip or knee replacement. J Bone Joint Surg [Am] 2001;83:336–45.
45. Kearon C, Hirsh J. Starting prophylaxis for venous thromboembolism postoperatively. Arch Intern Med 1995;155:366–72.
46. Hull RD, Brant RF, Pineo GF, et al. Preoperative vs postoperative initiation so low-molecular-weight heparin prophylaxis against venous thromboembolism in patients undergoing elective hip replacement. Arch Intern Med 1999;159:137–41.
47. Torholm C, Broeng L, Jorgensen PS, et al. Thromboprophylaxis by low-molecular-weight heparin in elective hip surgery. A placebo controlled study. J Bone Joint Surg [Br] 1991;73:434–8.
48. Francis CW, Pellegrini VD Jr, Totterman S, et al. Prevention of deep vein thrombosis after total hip arthroplasty: comparison of warfarin and dalteparin. J Bone Joint Surg [Am] 1997;79(9):1365–72.
49. Hull RD, Pineo GF, Francis C, et al. Low-molecular-weight heparin prophylaxis using dalteparin in close proximity to surgery vs. warfarin in hip arthroplasty patients. Arch Intern Med 2000;160:2199–207.
50. Hull RD, Pineo GF, Stein PD, et al. Timing of initial administration of low-molecular-weight heparin prophylaxis against deep vein thrombosis in patients following elective hip arthroplasty. Arch Intern Med 2001;161:1952–60.
51. Eriksson BI, Ekman S, Kalebo P, et al. Prevention of deep vein thrombosis after total hip replacement: direct thrombin inhibition with recombinant hirudin, CGP 39393. Lancet 1996;347:635–9.
52. Eriksson BI, Arfwidsson AC, Frison L, et al. A dose-ranging study of the oral direct thrombin inhibitor, ximelagatran, and its subcutaneous form, melagatran, compared with dalteparin in the prophylaxis of thromboembolism after hip or knee replacement: METHRO-1. Thromb Haemostasis 2002;87:231–7.
53. Eriksson BI, Bergqvist D, Kalebo P, et al. Melagatran for thrombin inhibition in orthopaedic surgery. Ximelagatran and melagatran compared with dalteparin for prevention of venous thromboembolism after total hip or knee replacement: the METHRO II randomized trial. Lancet 2002;360:1441–7.
54. Heit JA, Colwell CW, Francis CW, et al. AstraZeneca Arthroplasty Study Group: comparison of the oral direct thrombin inhibitor ximelagatran with enoxaparin as prophylaxis against venous thromboembolism after total knee replacement: a phase 2 dose-finding study. Arch Intern Med 2001;161:2215–21.
55. Colwell CW, Berkowitz SD, Davidson BL, et al. Comparison of ximelagatran, an oral direct thrombin inhibitor, with enoxaparin for the prevention of venous thromboembolism following total hip replacement. A randomized, double-blind study. J Thromb Haemost 2003;1(10):2119–30.
56. Turpie AGG, Gallus AS, Hoek JA, for the Pentasaccharide Investigators. A synthetic pentasaccharide for the prevention of deep-vein thrombosis after total hip replacement. N Engl J Med 2001;344:619–25.
57. Eriksson BI, Bauer KA, Lassen MR, et al. Fondaparinux compared with enoxaparin for the prevention of venous thromboembolism after hip-fracture surgery. N Engl J Med 2001;345:1298–304.
58. Bauer KA, Eriksson BI, Lassen MR, et al: Fondaparinux compared with enoxaparin for the prevention of venous thromboembolism after elective knee surgery. N Engl J Med 2001;345:1305–10.
59. Lassen MR, Bauer KA, Eriksson BI, et al. Postoperative fondaparinux versus preoperative enoxaparin for prevention of venous thromboembolism in elective

hip-replacement surgery: a randomised double-blind comparison. Lancet 2002;359: 1715–20.
60. Turpie AGG, Bauer KA, Eriksson BI, et al. Postoperative fondaparinux versus postoperative enoxaparin for prevention of venous thromboembolism after elective hip-replacement surgery: a randomised double-blind trial. Lancet 2002;359:1721–6.
61. Bounameaux H, Perneger T. Fondaparinux: a new synthetic pentasaccharide for thrombosis prevention. Lancet 2002;359:1710–11.
62. Dahl OE, Aspelin T, Arnesen H, et al. Increased activation of coagulation and formation of late deep venous thrombosis following discontinuation of thromboprophylaxis after hip replacement surgery. Thromb Res 1995;80:299–306.
63. White RH, Romano PS, Zhou H, et al. Incidence and time course of thromboembolic outcomes following total hip or knee arthroplasty. Arch Intern Med 1998;158:1525–31.
64. Hull RD, Pineo GF, Francis C, et al. Low-molecular-weight heparin prophylaxis using dalteparin extended out-of-hospital vs in-hospital warfarin/out-of-hospital placebo in hip arthroplasty patients. A double-blind, randomized comparison. Arch Intern Med 2000;160:2208–15.
65. Hull RD, Pineo GF, Stein PD, et al. Extended out-of-hospital low-molecular-weight heparin prophylaxis against deep venous thrombosis in patients after elective hip arthroplasty: a systematic review. Ann Intern Med 2001;135:858–869.
66. Samama CM, Vray M, Barre J, et al. Extended venous thromboembolism prophylaxis after total hip replacement: a comparison of low-molecular-weight heparin with oral anticoagulant. Arch Intern Med 2002;162:2191–6.
67. Prandoni P, Bruchi O, Sabbion P, et al. Prolonged thromboprophylaxis with oral anticoagulants after total hip arthroplasty: a prospective controlled randomized study. Arch Intern Med 2002;162(17):1966–71.
68. Eriksson BI, Lassen MR. Duration of prophylaxis against venous thromboembolism with fondaparinux after hip fracture surgery. Arch Intern Med 2003;163:1337.
69. Bergqvist D, Agnelli G, Cohen AT, et al. Duration of prophylaxis against venous thromboembolism with enoxaparin after surgery for cancer. N Engl J Med 2002;346:975–80.
70. Nicolaides AN, Breddin HK, Fareed J, et al. Prevention of venous thromboembolism. International Consensus Statement. Guidelines compiled in accordance with the scientific evidence. Int Angiol 2001;20:1–37.
71. Bergqvist D, Matzsch T, Burmark U, et al. Low molecular weight heparin given the evening before surgery compared with conventional low dose heparin in prevention of thrombosis. Br J Surg 1988;75:888–91.
72. Nurmohamed MT, Verhaeghe R, Haas S, et al. A comparative trial of a low molecular weight heparin (enoxaparin) versus standard heparin for the prophylaxis of postoperative deep vein thrombosis in general surgery. Am J Surg 1995;169:567–71.
73. ENOXACAN Study Group. Efficacy and safety of enoxaparin versus unfractionated heparin for prevention of deep vein thrombosis in elective cancer surgery: a double-blind randomized multicentre trial with venographic assessment. Br J Surg 1997;84:1099–103.
74. Leizorovicz A, Haugh MC, Chapuis FR, et al. Low molecular weight heparin in prevention of perioperative thrombosis. BMJ 1992;305:913–20.
75. Nurmohamed MT, Rosendaal FR, Buller HR, et al. Low-molecular-weight heparin versus standard heparin in general and orthopaedic surgery: a meta-analysis. Lancet 1992;340:152–6.
76. Koch A, Bouges S, Ziegler S, et al. Low molecular weight heparin and unfractionated heparin in thrombosis prophylaxis after major surgical intervention: update of previous meta-analyses. Br J Surg 1997;84:750–9.

77. Palmer AJ, Koppenhagen K, Kirchhof B, et al. Efficacy and safety of low molecular weight heparin, unfractionated heparin and warfarin for thrombo-embolism prophylaxis in orthopaedic surgery: a meta-analysis of randomised clinical trials. Haemostasis 1997;27:75–84.
78. Mismetti P, Laporte-Simitsidis S, Tardy B, et al. Prevention of venous thromboembolism in internal medicine with unfractionated or low-molecular-weight heparins: a meta-analysis of randomised clinical trials. Thromb Haemostasis 2000; 83:14–19.
79. Samama MM, Cohen AT, Darmon JY, et al. A comparison of enoxaparin with placebo for the prevention of venous thromboembolism in acutely ill medical patients. Prophylaxis in Medical Patients with Enoxaparin Study Group. N Engl J Med 1999;341:793–800.
80. Leizorovicz A, Cohen AT, Turpie AGG, et al. A randomized placebo controlled trial of dalteparin for the prevention of venous thromboembolism in 3706 acutely ill medical patients: the PREVENT medical thromboprophylaxis study. J Thromb Haemost 2003;1(suppl 1):abstract OC396.
81. Hillbom M, Erila T, Flosbach C, et al. Enoxaparin vs heparin for prevention of deep-vein thrombosis in acute ischaemic stroke: a randomized, double-blind study. Acta Neurol Scand 2002;106;84–92.
82. Geerts WH, Jay RM, Code KI, et al. A comparison of low dose heparin with low molecular weight heparin as prophylaxis against venous thromboembolism after major trauma. N Engl J Med 1996;335(10):701–7.
83. Ramos R, Salem BI, De Pawlikowski MP, et al. The efficacy of pneumatic compression stockings in the prevention of pulmonary embolism after cardiac surgery. Chest 1996;109(1):82–5.
84. Turpie AG, Delmore T, Hirsh J, et al. Prevention of venous thrombosis by intermittent sequential calf compression in patients with intracranial disease. Thromb Res Suppl 1979;15:611–16.
85. Skillman JJ, Collins RE, Coe NP, et al. Prevention of deep vein thrombosis in neurosurgical patients: a controlled, randomized trial of external pneumatic compression boots. Surgery (St Louis) 1978;83:354–8.
86. Hull RD, Raskob GE, Gent M, et al. Effectiveness of intermittent pneumatic leg compression for preventing deep vein thrombosis after total hip replacement. JAMA 1990;263:2313–17.
87. Francis CW, Pellegrini VD Jr, Marder VJ, et al. Comparison of warfarin and external pneumatic compression in prevention of venous thrombosis after total hip replacement. JAMA 1992;267(21):2911–15.
88. Hull RD, Delmore TJ, Hirsh J, et al. Effectiveness of intermittent pulsatile elastic stockings for the prevention of calf and thigh vein thrombosis in patients undergoing elective knee surgery. Thromb Res 1979;16:37–45.
89. McKenna R, Galante J, Bachmann F, et al. Prevention of venous thromboembolism after total knee replacement by high-dose aspirin or intermittent calf and thigh compression. Br Med J 1980;280:514–17.
90. Comerota AJ, Katz ML, White JV. Why does prophylaxis with external pneumatic compression for deep vein thrombosis fail? Am J Surg 1992;164:265–8.
91. Haddad FS, Kerry RM, McEwan JA, et al. Unanticipated variations between expected and delivered pneumatic compression therapy after elective hip surgery: a possible source of variation in reported patient outcomes. J Arthroplasty 2001;16:37–46.
92. Meyerowitz BR, Nelson R. Measurement of the velocity of blood in lower limb veins with and without compression surgery. Surgery (St Louis) 1964;56:481–6.

93. Sigel B, Edelstein AL, Felix WR Jr, et al. Compression of the deep venous system of the lower leg during inactive recumbency. Arch Surg 1973;106:38–43.
94. Wells PS, Lensing AWA, Hirsh J. Graduated compression stockings in the prevention of postoperative venous thromboembolism. A meta-analysis. Arch Intern Med 1994;154:67–72.
95. Francis CW, Pellegrini VD Jr, Leibert KM, et al. Comparison of two warfarin regimens in the prevention of venous thrombosis following total knee replacement. Thromb Haemostasis 1996;75:706–11.
96. Colwell CW Jr, Collis DK, Paulson R, et al. Comparison of enoxaparin and warfarin for the prevention of venous thromboembolic disease after total hip arthroplasty. J Bone Joint Surg [Am] 1999;81:932–40.
97. Paiement GD, Wessinger SJ, Waltman WC, et al. Low dose warfarin versus external pneumatic compression for prophylaxis against venous thromboembolism following total hip replacement. J Arthroplasty 1987;2:23–6.
98. Powers PJ, Gent M, Jay RM, et al. A randomized trial of less intense postoperative warfarin or aspirin therapy in the prevention of venous thromboembolism after surgery for fractured hip. Arch Intern Med 1989;149:771–4.
99. Poller L, McKernan A, Thomson JM, et al. Fixed minidose warfarin: a new approach to prophylaxis against venous thrombosis after major surgery. BMJ 1987;295:1309–12.
100. Hull RD, Pineo GF. A synthetic pentasaccharide for the prevention of deep-vein thrombosis. N Engl J Med 2001;345:291.
101. Eriksson BI, Agnelli G, Cohen AT, et al. The direct thrombin inhibitor melagatran followed by oral ximelagatran compared with enoxaparin for the prevention of venous thromboembolism after total hip or knee replacement: the EXPRESS study. J Thromb Haemost 2003;1(12):2490–6.
102. Francis CW, Berkowitz SD, Comp PC, et al. Comparison of ximelagatran with warfarin for the prevention of venous thromboembolism after total knee replacement. N Engl J Med. 2003;349(18):1703–12.

Subject Index